HOME FROM HOME

CYRIL DAVEY

HOME FROM HOME

The Story of
the Methodist Homes for the Aged

LONDON
EPWORTH PRESS

First published for
Methodist Homes for the Aged
by Epworth Press 1976

7162 0266 2

Made and printed in Great Britain
by The Garden City Press Limited
Letchworth, Hertfordshire SG6 1JS

Contents

Why?

Why a book about the Methodist Homes for the Aged?

I must admit that an out-of-the-blue telephone call from the Rev. Richard Connell, the General Secretary of the MHA—the abbreviation is sufficiently well-known to be acceptable—suggesting that I might write the story of the Methodist Homes produced nothing more from my end than an unenthusiastic agreement to think about it. It seemed that it could hardly help being dull—an account of old buildings and old bones. In fact, as soon as I began to assemble material and, more, to visit the homes, the project became increasingly exciting.

I knew something of the MHA already. My mother had been a resident and neither she nor I could speak more highly of the care she had received and the fellowship she had shared. In the home where she lived I had seen some of the problems and the achievements of a staff which was always stretched to do the work adequately, and yet never ceased to do it with love and understanding.

I was not unacquainted with some of the other homes, too. Yet how could such a book avoid being a catalogue of houses, a balance-sheet of money raised hardly and spent, for the most part judiciously if apparently, in more recent years, lavishly? This last impression was to change, too. But so did my whole approach. The buildings are incidental, for this is a story of *people*. People with insight, vision and dedication. People giving service in unthought-of ways. People in need, finding new hope and new life. Old people who remain young in heart, and others who regain youth in outlook. People waiting on long lists with the hope of ending their days not so much in comfort, still less in luxury, as in the company of others like themselves. People, at every level of this heart-warming organization, whose only concern is to serve others.

This transformation of what might have been a chore into a privilege in which I have rejoiced and been humbled, has not come from reading minutes, memos or letters, but through visiting each one of the homes. Many of them my wife has visited with me—and has asked more penetrating questions than I could have thought of raising. We have been profoundly moved by the courage, initiative, interests and creativeness of the elderly people to whom we talked, and who showed us their rooms, their cherished possessions and their handiwork. We have been impressed, though not surprised, by the selfless devotion, individual care and interest of matrons, assistants and resident and daily staff. We have been careful to visit kitchens, staff quarters and vegetable-gardens, as well as to look at lounges and rose-beds! Everywhere we were welcomed, and we deeply appreciated it.

I must express my gratitude to those without whose help this book could not have been written. This includes residents and staff, the headquarters staff of the MHA, and many others. To try to detail them all would be impossible. But I must make two special acknowledgements. First, to my friend Reg Spray, who has served as Administrator at Westminster and travelled ceaselessly round the country for two decades in the service of the elderly. He went to immense trouble to provide material for which I asked—and his wife was as busy as he was in reducing tapes, memos and memories into typescript. My second debt is to a group of men, all highly individualistic, some retired ministers but mostly laymen, each highly skilled, without whom the Homes could not function. *These are the local treasurers for each home*. The word is a misnomer which grossly limits and undervalues the service they give. They are, indeed, the local 'administrators'. True, they collect the residents' payments! But in many cases they are to be found in the homes four or five days a week. They are confidants of the residents, helping to solve personal, family and occasionally financial problems. They are the mainstay of the local Home Committee and the springboard for action about repairs, maintenance, improvements and emergency needs. They are complementary to the matron and work with her. They provide an important link with the local community and, because they are themselves local men, produce a long-term element of continuity as members of staff come and go. Their word is not law, and they would not wish it to be, but it carries great weight with the headquarters at Westminster, for whom they are the representative in the local home. No tribute would do them more than justice.

What, then, is the over-all impression of one who has had the privilege of seeing so much of the homes at close quarters and comparing the present reality with the first visions of people like the Rev. Walter Hall, Sir George Martin and Mrs Hilda Bartlett Lang—the first their pioneer, the other two the chairman and treasurer for thirty years?

In simple terms, this. The Methodist Homes for the Aged provide unquestionably the most significant contribution of the Methodist Church to society and community in this century. In planning for them, and in going far beyond the early dreams about them, they are the counterpart of Methodism's other great social contribution in the last century, the National Children's Home.

Yet to end there would imply that we were going to look at an organization. The truth is far more intimate and personal. It was summed up by an eighty-year-old resident, after more than ten years in one of the homes.

'When I write to my friends I always spell it with a small "h" —because, you see, it isn't a "Home" at all . . . it's just "home".'

The 1930s

Ground plan

'The one quality of which the aged should never be robbed is self-respect.'

1

'Don't let me go to the Union!'

The room in a back-street in Tottenham was small, untidy and had a none-too-clean smell. That was not surprising, since its occupant was an elderly woman whom life had used hardly. Her husband had died in World War I. Her children had left home and only her daughter came to see her occasionally. Aged sixty-five, she looked ten years older because of under-nourishment and a nagging pain for which a doctor with too long a list of poor patients gave her little but a brusque word of sympathy. With next to no money and little strength she did her feeble best to bring some sort of order to her few cherished possessions about the room. Her bed, with a thin sheet, was without a cover and almost without a mattress.

There were hundreds of rooms like this in Tottenham, and tens of thousands all over London. They were to be found in every town in Britain, and few villages did not possess their rural counterpart. But it was not the poverty, the hunger or the squalor which was the real degradation. It was that, because few seemed to care about such people, they lost even their own self-respect. They were statistics in papers published by research writers. They provided vivid paragraphs in election manifestos. But, as individuals, they scarcely existed. The tragedy was too common for headlines even when they died alone and were only discovered days, or weeks, later.

To say that *nobody* cared was sometimes inaccurate. The one occasional bright spot—much more welcome than the apparently inhuman rent-collector—was a visit from the vicar, the priest or the local minister. It was to the minister in Tottenham that the frail woman, old ten years too soon, made her anguished appeal.

'I can't stay on here; there's no money for the rent. And I've got nowhere to go . . . nowhere at all. But please, Mr Hall—*don't let them take me to the Union!*'

'The Union'—the universal word for the workhouse—was the dread, and all too often the inevitable end, of the poor and especially of the aged.

The minister, sitting on the one rickety chair, had no answer. For *this* woman it would *have* to be the workhouse. There was nowhere else to go.

Occasions like that happened too often for a man like Walter Hall, the Methodist minister in Tottenham, to be unaffected by them even though he could do nothing to change the situation. Another pressure, on the same subject, came from the politicians. Tottenham was an over-crowded, under-employed, under-privileged area of North London. Its people and its politicians tended to be Labour. Moderate by modern radical standards, its MPs were regarded by the better-off, by the various 'establishments', and not least by the Church, as dangerous people who wanted to undermine the secure foundations of society. For their part they had little sympathy with the lethargic middle-classes and, in the main, no liking or respect for the Church.

'You're in a safe job. You've never been unemployed, and you don't know what it feels like to wonder where the next meal will come from—or even if there will be one. The Church is just a way of escaping from the realities of life.' The tirade was familiar to Walter Hall, socially-conscious as he was. So was the denunciation he had heard scores of times from his local politicians. 'What is the Church doing for the poor?'

It would have been simple, and accurate, to reply: 'As much as many of the politicians!'

The riposte might have scored a debating point but it dodged the issue. The Church, in truth, offered a little help to the few, but nowhere near enough. Still less did it challenge society as a whole to take its responsibilities seriously. And that was something that worried Hall as he went about his daily pastoral work and pondered in his study at home. For him, the Church and its ministry ensured security . . . he imagined how he would have felt, in the depressed 1930s, had that security been removed.

The Rev. Walter Hall, pioneer and key-figure of the Methodist Homes for the Aged, was born in Nottingham in 1876. He entered the ministry of what was then the United Methodist Free Churches, in 1905. After college he went for two years to Jamaica, but thirty-eight of his forty-year ministry were spent in England, and half of them in London. His last fifteen years were in Tottenham and it was there, more than anywhere else, that the plight of the aged was thrust on him. On the surface he was cool, efficient and meticulous, and his carefully detailed administration led to his appointment as secretary of the London North Methodist District and, later, as its chairman—the equivalent of a diocesan bishop. No one held office of this sort without a certain toughness, a far-sighted determination to hold his course however rough the passage. He belonged to a generation of Methodist administrators who knew their law-books, their own capacities and their districts very well indeed. They also knew what they wanted, and more often than not they achieved it.

Some of these qualities are essential to men and women who see visions and are adamant that they shall not fade in the harsh light of reality. But, where those visions concern people, other characteristics are equally needed—and Walter Hall had them to the full. A passionate sense of justice; an anger with systems and people who deny rights to the poor, the infirm and the oppressed; a love of people; and, above all, a deep personal awareness of God who had revealed his own love for men and women in Jesus Christ—these were displayed throughout his ministry and, long after he retired, to the end of his long life.

It was the conjunction of these qualities, together with his experience as a minister amongst the poor, that caused him such unease when he was attacked about the relative indifference of the Church, to those in need. He was not, after all, only the minister of a local church. He held a responsible position under the Methodist Conference. He spoke with authority for, and to, the Church.

The agonized appeal, local for him but repeated all over the country in town and village, refused to be dismissed.

'Please—don't let them take me to the Union!'

Almost from its very beginnings the Christian Church had a special concern for the sick, the aged and the poor. Jesus himself had often turned his back on the privileged to minister to the rejected, and his most biting parable proclaimed that heaven was only for those who gave themselves to people in need. By the third century Christian institutions had been established for the aged, the sick and the helpless poor. By the sixth century they had spread to Italy and France, challenging the ruthless cruelty of old faiths as Christ conquered the old gods. Love in action became the hallmark of the Christian.

In the Middle Ages the monasteries took over the same task. 'Hospitals' were places where the Church offered 'hospitality' to the poor as well as to the sick. The indigent 'infirm' gave their name to the 'infirmaries' and, with the almshouses, were places of temporary shelter and relief for the traveller. At the convent gate there was often a daily distribution of bread.

Perhaps the most notable, as well as the earliest, home for the aged run by the Church in Britain is still active and can be visited. The tourist at Winchester Cathedral has only to walk a few steps to find the entrance to the Hospital of St Cross. Generations of almsmen have lived here since it was founded in 1136, less than a century after the Norman conquest of England. Still existing for men only, the visitor will be shown round by one of the Brethren. As he looks at the gate where a loaf and two pints of rough wine were given to all who called, or at the place where men have worshipped for 800 years, or is welcomed into one of the small rooms where these men live in private contentment, he will be transported back to a time when the Church was the only institution to have a true concern for the poverty-stricken and the old.

Small and scattered though such charity was, it could be found all over Britain and it only ceased, in the main, when Henry VIII dissolved the monasteries in the sixteenth century, giving the buildings as rewards or bribes to his favourites, and stealing their gold, their jewels, their precious possessions and their money to replenish his own almost empty treasury. Two things, amongst many others, resulted from Henry's pillaging of the Church. The first was the end, not only of the monastic establishments, but of the hospitals which had been one of their more praiseworthy activities. The other was the beginnings of the Poor Law in England.

'Charity', that gracious New Testament word for love in action, was quickly to become a cold, despised and hated term for a heartless and often cruel system of administrative relief.

The legal intention was fair enough—to provide work for those who could not find it, to 'discourage idlenesss', and to protect society as a whole against unscrupulous 'rogues and vagabonds' who knew the easiest way to live was to beg and sometimes the most obvious was to steal. In 1576 an Act was passed which provided for 'abiding places' where the poor who were prepared to work could find some sort of shelter. For the wealthy there was pleasure and privilege; for the poor, there was never enough food, work or wages. True, many of the wealthy had a genuine piety and some sort of social conscience. Acts were passed under Elizabeth I which both encouraged and protected bequests for charity, and the Poor Law of 1601 included a great deal that remains today the basis of modern Charity Law under which the present Methodist Homes, as well as thousands of other charities, are able to operate effectively, without hindrance and indeed with valuable concessions.

It is an astonishing fact that from the middle of the fifteenth century to the beginning of the seventeenth over £3,000,000 was set apart by private individuals as charitable bequests for the foundation of colleges, grammar schools and almshouses. In its modern equivalent it is an immense sum and shows a genuine Christian concern for the poor, since the schools and colleges were intended to benefit boys of ability whose parents were without adequate means. Most of the almshouses were related to parish churches, with governors appointed by the church, and were meant for needy residents of the parish itself.

But alongside this generosity of spirit there existed a much less sensitive provision for those in need. Few children were able to go to a charity school, and still fewer of the old could find room in an almshouse. For those who otherwise might have died without shelter there was often a single building, provided out of public funds, where the young and the old, the sick, the infirm and the blind, the destitute, the homeless and the mentally ill were herded together in squalor and superintended with the utmost harshness by illiterate and sadistic overseers. This building was the 'workhouse'—for even the young, the deranged and the feeble aged could hardly expect to eat unless they worked! Only the labourer was worthy of his coarse bread and his dirty straw pallet. 'Workhouse', then, was an apt description. It was used, perhaps for the first time, in Colchester in 1594 and was in common usage from the beginning of the next century.

Some sort of 'relief' was often available to those who could not find room even in the workhouse—and there was never enough room for those who needed even that disgusting shelter. But, at the beginning of the last century, there were widespread riots over the way 'relief' was doled out. They resulted in transportation for life for several hundred labourers, but at least they made the government look afresh at the cost of public relief and the provision for those needing aid. It became evident that too much attention was being given to the able-bodied and too little to the aged.

So what was needed? The Victorians saw only one answer. There must be more workhouses, at immense cost to the state and the local authorities. In the middle of the century Florence Nightingale's demand for an adequate nursing service was heard with extravagant horror. To work amongst the sick, the poor or the unwashed aged was viewed as degradation by a generation which opposed Lord Shaftesbury's attack on the use of women and children in the mines, and was affronted by Charles Kingley's 'tract for the times', *The Water Babies*, which exposed the shocking plight of small boys used as chimney-sweeps. It needed the popular novels of Charles Dickens, with their horrifying delineation of the anguish of the poor, to stir the lethargy of the nation.

Society as a whole insulated and excused itself. Poverty was 'their own fault' or 'the fault of their families'. A measure of judicious harshness and the reward of 'bread for work' would bring people to their senses! In the 1830s, 643 regional Unions replaced the thousands of small administrative units responsible for the poor and aged all over Britain. Between 1830 and 1840 hundreds of new workhouses were built by these regional Unions—and the workhouse itself became commonly and bitterly known as 'the Union'. By 1840 the average workhouse contained more than 200 inmates. People of all kinds continued to be herded together. Dickens's *Oliver Twist*, stripped of its colourful staging and its Lionel Bart music, is less of a caricature and more of a literal description than we like to realize.

The strait-jacket, the cell, the exercise yard, the meagre ration of bread, the vicious overseer, the drab serge uniform—these continued to be the marks of the workhouse until well into the twentieth century. Any townsman or villager born in Queen Victoria's glorious reign had good reason to be afraid of living too long or of being rejected by his or her family.

It is almost impossible to re-create the horror of the workhouse *—and still more incredible that they were the main, and indeed almost the only, refuge for the aged when World War II ended in 1945.*

Not until the beginning of this century was much discrimination made amongst the 'inmates' of the workhouse, though officially there was a distinction between 'deserving old people' of 'blameless character' and the 'undeserving poor'. Where this distinction existed the 'deserving' were housed in separate dormitories and day-rooms from the 'undeserving'. They could occasionally visit friends and could even go to church. But, well into the century, only 1,000 of the 140,000 elderly people in workhouses had such 'privileges'.

Anyone who can remember visiting the local 'Union' in the 1930s will have a grim recollection of ugly and utilitarian buildings. There were three or four storeys, reached by narrow staircases. The wards were narrow, poorly lit by windows placed high in the walls, and the dormitories were sickeningly overcrowded. Some wards had 100 beds, each less than two feet from its neighbour. There were no lockers, no privacy, no personal belongings. The day-rooms were large, cheerless, and filled with aimless, often senile, figures slumped into, or slipping out of, small hard chairs. The rules were restrictive and generally harshly administered. Wardens and orderlies seldom conceived of their charges as real people who might, in some cases, respond to humane treatment. Gentleness and compassion were rare, in most institutions.

By 1946 the number of aged people in workhouses in Britain, or in workhouses which had been turned into hospitals for the senile or the chronic sick, was greater than in 1900.

This was the background to the life of the poor, and especially the aged poor, as Walter Hall ministered in Tottenham in the 1930s.

2

'Somebody should do something!'

It is one of the world's most dangerous phrases.

Say it in the committee meeting of any organization and the response—if any comes at all—is predictable. 'Well, why don't *you* do it?'

Many of the most far-reaching pioneer efforts and the most splendidly effective organizations have come about through that phrase, and that response. For the Christian to say that somethings needs doing is at once to become vulnerable. There is always the chance that God will utter his own urgent command—'Go and do it!'

So it was with Walter Hall.

The need was obvious and desperate, though the likelihood of doing anything far-reaching was remote. But the possibility could not be evaded. He could only obey the prompting of God and his own heart. He must do *something*.

He decided to use his position as one of Methodism's district chairmen to call together a group of interested people for a discussion of the situation. Before he began, to avoid a debate without any clear parameters, he set out to see what possibilities existed. Few of those who attended that gathering in 1937 are still alive, but the general line of the meeting is remembered. Walter Hall himself directed it, for he alone knew what was in his mind. He outlined the drastic situation of old people as he saw it. Help on a large scale he believed to be the responsibility of government and the local authorities, and necessary changes in the inhuman conditions under which tens of thousands of old people had to exist was too big a task for voluntary workers. But there was *one* thing they could do.

The real point of the meeting, Hall explained, was that within Methodism itself were many elderly people who could no longer look after themselves adequately. Not all were poor, but too many could not afford proper food or heating, and fell ill as a consequence. In some cases they had no family; in others, as everyone knew, families could not or would not look after them.

'Many of these good people have been loyal servants of the Church and of their Lord. They have a right to expect that the Church they love and have served faithfully should not turn away from them in their old age.'

The little group stirred, nodded their heads—but had an uneasy awareness that they might find themselves committed to action before they realized it.

'We must do something about it . . . *now*! I want your support in a scheme to find a house which we can use as a home for some of these people. It won't be easy. The time is not ripe for this sort of adventure. And it will cost money. . . . Are you prepared to back such a plan?'

There was a good deal of discussion, but Hall had no doubt of the outcome. He was given encouragement to continue planning, to try to find a house and to call the informal committee together again when he had found what he wanted. But, as their trains thundered or dawdled across the countryside, the committee members wondered what they had done. Walter Hall was always persuasive—passionate in his commitment to social justice and shrewd in getting his way with a committee. But, away from that convincing presence, the difficulties loomed larger than he had admitted. Local demands were heavy on church members. The memory of the great depression was still all too vivid; only a few years had passed since the weary, grey procession of the unemployed had tramped slowly to London from all over the country to demand action from the government.

Surely this was the wrong time to initiate a scheme so tenuously based?

To Walter Hall the difficulties were very real, too, and he did not minimize them. Hitler's voice echoed stridently from the 'wireless', and the disposition to treat him as a cartoon joke was being dissipated by events, though the British government appeared to believe that if he were treated like a gentleman our own shores would be safe. Mussolini was swaggering his way towards the ruthless conquest of Abyssinia. Russia hung over the eastern horizon like a cloud that might herald a storm or disappear before the sunshine of optimism. In the general climate of unreality which pervaded the nation Hall went out to look at a property which might serve his purpose.

He did not go into the streets of London without a proper sense of direction. He had served in Brixton before going to Tottenham. Wandsworth was not far from Brixton—and by Wandsworth Common there might well be the very thing he had in mind.

Before the three divided Methodist Churches were reunited in 1932 the old United Methodist Church, of which he had been a minister, had its own Order of Deaconesses. In 1903 it had been given a house at Wandsworth to serve as the headquarters of the Order. When Methodist Union was consummated the United Methodist Deaconess Order was merged with the larger one in the Wesleyan Methodist Church, which had been started by Dr T. B. Stephenson, founder of the National Children's Home. The Wesleyans had their own training centre and Deaconess House at Ilkley, in Yorkshire, and since 1932 the Wandsworth House had not been used for its original purpose. It was this house, 32 Bolingbroke Grove, at Wandsworth Common, that Walter Hall had had in mind even before the first committee was called together, though he had been shrewd enough not to disclose all his plans at the first meeting.

The second committee, somewhat different in personnel from the first, responded with caution to Hall's enthusiasm and to his report on the house. The political scene had darkened. Hitler had marched into Czechoslovakia. Austria was in his grasp. His claim that he had 'no further territorial claim in Europe' was manifestly incredible when it was backed with the might of the German army and air force. In Germany the small Confessional Church was under pressure because of its opposition to Hitler's political views and his racial violence. The Jews were being systematically exterminated. At such a time, said the committee, who could hope to raise money to buy and equip a home for a few elderly Methodists?

Walter Hall watched his committee depart, acknowledging that they were probably right.

On Sunday, 3rd September 1939, as he began to lead his congregation in worship, the air-raid sirens sounded for the first time. Chamberlain's dry pedantic voice was broadcast to the nation.

Britain had declared war on Germany.

The 1940s

The Foundations are laid

'The best Physicians are Doctor Diet,
Doctor Quiet and Doctor Merryman.'
—*Jonathan Swift*

3

The real beginning

'The Conference WILL *Meet!'*

In June 1943 the *Methodist Recorder* carried the news on its front page, and to not a few Methodist's the sub-editor's headline had a ring of biblical assurance. The annual Conference of the Methodist Church is an administrative and legal assembly of great authority, but then it also appeared as a symbol of stability and continuity. Its cancellation—and there had been talk of it—would almost have implied capitulation to the enemy.

It was a dark hour in British history. Two years earlier, after Dunkirk, Hitler had proclaimed 'a war of annihilation' against his enemies. The City of London had been set ablaze and Buckingham Palace bombed. Coventry, Merseyside, Southampton and Birmingham had been blitzed before the year had ended, and Cardiff and Plymouth had suffered the same terror in the first few weeks of 1941. The Nazi invasion of Britain had been deferred because of the gallantry of 'the Few' who fought out the aerial 'Battle of Britain', but with rationing, the black-out and bad news from the war areas everything was in short supply except courage. At the end of 1941, following the bombing of the American fleet at Pearl Harbour and the entry of both Japan and the USA into the war, Asia and the Pacific had become new battle-grounds of continental proportions. The incredible fall of Singapore highlighted Japanese imperial strength; much of Asia had been over-run; the Pacific islands were occupied or being fought over. In Europe there were few signs of Germany weakening, and North Africa was dominated by the German and Italian armies. The fall of Tobruk, on the Egyptian frontier, seemed to herald yet further disasters. Only determination, optimism and the speeches of Winston Churchill promised an outcome favourable to Britain. Even if the allies 'won the war' the devastation in

Britain was incalculable. Private homes and, amongst public buildings, Methodist churches had suffered greatly.

Yet Methodism continued its life and did not lose its spirit, either of faith or service. The Conference met in Birmingham Central Hall in July 1943, in a city which showed the ravages of old and new air attacks. Dr Leslie Church was in the presidential chair and a new secretary of the Conference, Edwin Finch, was controlling the business for the first time. It was his duty to arrange the order of business for the week. In general, the least important matters came last—and, in the morning of the last day of the Conference, he had included an item remitted from the previous year. Its description was 'Eventide Homes'.

Some things about the previous Conference in Manchester were vividly remembered. There had been, for instance, a sharp debate about 'dancing on Methodist premises', with an unforgetable interjection from the octogenarian Dr Scott Lidgett. 'I went to a party . . . I even danced with a lady . . . she was not demoralised . . . but three minutes was enough!' Most representatives could recall that interlude—but not what had been said about 'Eventide Homes'.

When Walter Hall ascended the tribune to speak on that final morning it was evident that, however much destruction had been wreaked on British cities, his own 'castle in the clouds' remained intact. It must have seemed no more material than that. Fortunately the text of the previous year's resolution was printed in the *Agenda.* The 1942 Conference had appointed a small committee, with Walter Hall as convenor,

> 'to consider the advisability and practicability of establishing Methodist Homes for people usually of sixty years of age or over, who desire to avail themselves of such amenities as the Homes provide, and agree to contribute to their support according to their means.'

Hall's committee had met during the year to clarify their hopes, establish practical grounds for them and try to ensure their support by the Conference. In the 'democracy' of Methodism, where the annual Conference exercised absolute authority, the official blessing, or at least sanction, of the Conference was essential if the idea were to be carried forward.

The principal means of informing the Methodist public of what the Conference discussed was the *Methodist Recorder*, but in 1942 it had not even mentioned the discussion on 'Eventide Homes'. To those who happened to hear of it, it must have sounded a cranky and idealistic notion put forward at completely the wrong moment. The reporter for the last morning of the 1943 Conference at Birmingham, squeezing a paragraph or so into the end of his final column, did little to clarify his readers' hazy knowledge. It is hard to believe that the report accurately reflected what was said, though no other public record exists.

'The Rev. Walter Hall', he wrote, 'reported on the work of the committee set up the previous year. He said there were some aged Methodists in other homes, though these homes had long waiting lists. He explained that the committee's desire was not to establish separate houses so much as "hostels to accommodate twenty or more persons".' (It seems unlikely that Hall used the word 'hostels'!) 'The need might be met by "allowing people to furnish their own homes in various parts of the country" with a maximum of privacy on a basis of self-maintenance.'

The reporting, or the sub-editing, was to say the least inadequate. But it is not surprising. *The proposals, in fact, envisaged a revolutionary and almost completely new concept in the provision of care for the aged.*

Some of the other matters which Hall raised were reported more clearly.

'We want to encourage local initiative. This is not just a matter for a London committee. There is no reason why districts and circuits should not establish homes of this kind themselves.

'Those whom we expect to receive in the Homes will be Methodists for the most part, but members of other churches who are in need and are of good character, will not be excluded.

'The Conference may well ask: what about "ways and means"? I can only say that a good many friends who know about what we propose have written and offered their support. But we cannot take their money, however much we need it, until the Conference has agreed that we go forward. We want this to be an *official* action of the Conference, not the activity of a few interested individuals.' The future development of the Homes was to show how wise was Hall's insistence on this principle.

'The committee would be very grateful if someone would present us with the first house!'

Many members of the Conference had already left, but amongst those who remained there were growls of approval (this assembly never claps and seldom shouts) and some murmurs of incomprehension. The secretary of the Conference was, by this time, attuned to its moods.

'Have the members of the Conference actually *read* the report which is printed in the *Agenda*?' It was a good question. He put the position firmly. 'We must not act without thinking. If the Conference agrees you must understand that it will involve giving the committee the power to establish homes of this kind almost immediately.'

There was a sudden flurry of discussion. A legacy existed—but it must be taken up within three years, and the man had already been dead for twelve months. A knowledgeable layman pointed out that it would only bring in £150 a year. It was better to move slowly than to act precipitately for the sake of £150.

The aged dancer, Dr Lidgett, intervened. It was not necessary to debate every point in the committee's report or Mr Hall's suggestions. Surely the Conference could give the whole idea its blessing? Let them give their general approval and ask for another report next year.

Suddenly anxious to be finished with the matter and go home the Conference agreed, with unexpected warmth. Hall sat out the remainder of the business and went out into the war-torn world, where houses were being destroyed daily in every part of Britain, and set off for London.

Though he was still chairman of the London North District he had moved south of the city with his invalid wife, and settled at Selsdon, near Croydon. Arriving at home he found that the local minister, Garfield Curnow, and his wife were having tea with Mrs Hall. Hall did not even pause to hang up his coat but marched straight in on them. As he did so he flung his arms high, beaming with enthusiasm and happiness.

'We've won.' Then, before they had time to ask questions, he went on, 'The Conference has given us permission to go ahead with the Homes!'

For the moment, that was enough. There would be more difficulties than even he had imagined. Some of his hopes would not be fulfilled, others would change, and many of the details would be modified. But none of that spilled over into the Selsdon sitting-room. He could hardly contain his excitement or wait to start moving with his friends in what might well prove the disheartening business of finding the first house. The summer that followed was filled with work, much of it unrelated to the Homes. There was correspondence with the members of his committee but, in the main, his task was still the two-fold responsibility of caring for his own church at Tottenham and overseeing his District. In assessing Hall's pioneer role it must never be forgotten that the Homes were something quite extra to his already heavy workload. It would have been impossible without the practical encouragement of a group of far-seeing friends. Some were ministers who had been his colleagues and close confidants through the years; not a few were laymen whose professional skills and wide range of contacts were to be invaluable. It was one of these, Charles Hulbert, who had long been involved in the evangelistic and social work of the central halls, who made a suggestion of great consequence.

Hulbert had for many years known and been given great support by Joseph Rank, the millionaire Methodist mill-owner, and he knew how deep was the commitment to Methodism of some of Rank's family. One was his son Arthur, later to become Lord Rank, and another his daughter Hilda, married to a minister who had always worked in the 'mission' areas of the Church's life, Fred Bartlett Lang.

'Why don't you ask Mrs Lang to be treasurer of the Homes?' asked Hulbert.

He was not the only one with this idea. A well-known Yorkshire layman, Sir George Martin, had been interested in the idea of the Homes almost from its inception. One day Sir George and Mrs Lang were talking about the work in which they were both interested.

'Of course you'll be chairman', said Mrs Lang.

Sir George had his answer ready. 'Provided you'll be the treasurer', he replied.

In July 1944 Hall reported to the Conference which met at Oxford Place Chapel in Leeds. Once more the Homes came last in the business of the Conference, but Hall now had some very positive things to say.

Following the general approval given the previous year the committee had been exploring practical possibilities. It had bought its first house, and this was a promising beginning. But even if they had twenty homes the stream of applications proved there would be more than enough people to fill them. The letters appealing to be accepted as residents were heart-rending. Few people realized how deep and widespread was the need, in every part of the country. Their paramount requirement, now, was money. He had come to the Conference with the intention of asking it to agree that a large capital fund be set up. The amount in the committee's mind was £50,000.

There was a buzz throughout the large chapel, filled with representatives and visitors. The sum seemed immense, especially when houses could be bought for a few thousands of pounds. True, the allied invasion of Europe had begun, but nobody imagined the end of the war immediately in sight. There were rumours of worse bombing to come—and, indeed, the 'flying bombs' were to be ravaging London within a couple of months. How much money it would take to rebuild or repair the hundreds of churches and halls already damaged or destroyed it was impossible to estimate. Surely, said those representatives from the deeply-scarred areas of Britain to each other, this was no time to be asking for £50,000, however sympathetic they might feel.

Walter Hall was continuing, persuasive but well aware of the reluctance he had to overcome. His next words were dramatic. 'I think we should revise the committee's request for £50,000', he went on. 'I have had, within the last day or so, a letter offering £15,000 if we set the final total at *£60,000*.

The letter had come from Mrs Lang, though he did not disclose that fact, and the 'challenge offer' from the Joseph Rank

Benevolent Trust, set up by Rank to perpetuate his generosity to his beloved Methodist church.

The mood of the Conference changed swiftly, from caution to enthusiasm.

More securely than in the previous year, the day was won. The resolutions proposed by Hall were carried without argument. The authority of the committee was established and, in the final resolution, a change of title was included. The Conference directed

> 'that from time to time as and when the Conference thinks fit, homes to be known as "Methodist Homes for the Aged" be established by or with the approval of the Conference and in such places as the Conference shall approve.'

The new committee included thirteen ministers and fourteen laymen. Amongst them were ministers who were to mean a good deal in the years that followed—Lorne Cornish, Charles Hulbert, Robinson Whittaker, George Taylor and William Stoate were some of them. The lay members were just as significant; some, like F. Johnston Carey and Mrs Elsie Hill, for instance, would have their own place in the actual building projects that were to come. Inevitable nominations were 'Mrs F. Bartlett Lang as Treasurer and the Rev. Walter Hall as Convenor'. The name 'Sir George Martin, K.B.E.', however, set in the alphabetical order of the committee, gave no indication of the invaluable part he was to play in the future.

Now, incontestably, the Methodist Homes for the Aged had ceased to be a private enthusiasm or a committee's baby which might or might not grow to maturity, and had become by the will of the Conference the responsibility of the whole Methodist Church. No one could foretell its future, and whether it might succeed or founder. Few would have dared to prophesy how many homes it would have, how many people it would be serving, or what the pattern of that service might be in thirty years' time, even if it then existed.

Nor, probably, did Sir George Martin or Mrs Hilda Lang imagine that there would be thirty years of unremitting and dedicated work before they would finally hand over their tasks as chairman and treasurer. Britain, after all, was still at war. A house had been bought but money had still to be raised. A desperate need had been exposed but the main response had been requests for help rather than promises of support. A small beginning—a very small one—had been made. It is time to go behind the public façade of the Conference and see what had been achieved and what was being planned.

4

'The Evening Chair'

Wallington

Joseph Rank, though he died the year before the Leeds Conference gave full approval to the Homes, is in a real sense part of their story. It was through the generous stimulus of the trust fund he established that not a little of its work was made possible. More significantly, it was in large measure through his daughter that a meticulous stewardship was exercised in the use of the slim budget of the early days and, throughout her years as treasurer, in the building, equipment and maintenance of the homes. Her personal qualities, as well as her financial ability to support the work generously—though always privately—owed a great deal to her father.

It was in a windmill-cottage on the Holderness road in Hull that Joseph Rank was born in 1854. Though his father's flour was highly regarded for its quality, there were more than the wind and the occasional poor harvest to contend with; over twenty other windmills could be seen from the balcony of the Rank mill. Competition for trade was vigorous. Joseph himself was regarded by his father as slow, lacking in initiative and energy, and too irresponsible to run the business on his father's death. In his will he appointed trustees to watch over the mill and his widow's interests, and bequeathed Joseph £500 of the £30,000 he left. That was in 1874.

Within ten years Joseph Rank had worked so hard in his own rented mill that he changed from the old mill-stones turned by sails to a new process, and established a 'rolling-mill' with steel rollers that would produce twelve sacks of flour an hour. Though he then had to collect orders by pony-trap each day, and his only assistants were two young men with no experience in milling, the business grew fast. By 1891 he established the Clarence mill on the river Humber. It was the beginning of a new era of prosperity for the city. Rank himself, already a rich man, bought Willersley House in the Hull suburb of Pearson Park. At the beginning of the century he moved to London, to Bushey Down on Tooting Common.

Though his evangelical experience—in Methodist terms, his conversion—did not change his tough, competitive, commercial spirit, it affected his personal life deeply and, in particular, induced in him a responsible attitude to the use of his constantly increasing wealth. His service as a Sunday-school teacher, begun in Hull and continued in London, lasted for more than fifty years. He was passionately evangelical, with a simple personal faith, and he believed that 'central halls' and 'missions' would attract working-people who were unlikely to enter the conventional and conservative churches. By the outbreak of World War I his mills were established in Ireland as well as England and he was on the way to being one of the richest men in Europe —yet he seldom missed the Monday night devotional 'class meeting' at Tooting.

His character, simple in his religious attitudes, was complex as he matched 'getting the most out of his works and workers' with astonishing personal generosity. No detail of his expenditure was too trivial to be scrutinized, but he would support without reserve a project in which he believed. Yet, at the same time, he always tried to avoid personal credit for his giving. Though Methodism as a whole knew him to be the constant 'Anonymous Donor' to home and overseas mission he never allowed his name to be mentioned.

It was typical of his approach to his money that, for many years, he met the deficit on the Methodist Missionary Society's annual accounts, but always anonymously. Between 1920 and 1939 his gifts to that Society totalled £1,136,687. Then, nearly eighty years old, he gave in trust to the Missionary Society shares worth over £1,250,000.

At about the same time, to ensure that Methodism would continue to benefit from his wealth after his death as it had done during his lifetime, he established the Joseph Rank Benevolent Trust from which gifts have poured munificently into almost every circuit in Methodism, and into many of its special projects, since his death in 1943.

It was in such a family that his daughter Hilda grew up, seeing and sharing the warmth of her father's nature as well as his shrewdness and punctilious stewardship over money.

Born in Hull, she lived at Willersley House—a name that was later to feature in the history of the MHA. At Southport, where she was a boarder at Wintersdorf school, she recalls that two prim mistresses referred to her as 'this wild child'—the daughter of a man who had made his own way and who, in turn, wanted *her* own way. But she grew into a Christian faith and experience that was all her own, and came to love Methodism and what it stood for as much as her father had done.

It was at an annual meeting of the Methodist Conference in Plymouth that a friend introduced her to a quiet, good-looking young minister and left them talking. She reported, many years later, what happened.

'What did you think of him?' her friend asked.

Looking back on that moment she commented: 'I wasn't going to tell *her* what I thought—but I married him!'

The young minister was Fred Bartlett Lang, and out of that first meeting came a happy and loving home with a family of girls and one boy, the youngest, Paul, who was eventually to succeed his father as the secretary of the Joseph Rank Benevolent Trust.

After five years in Bristol Bartlett Lang spent the remainder of his ministry in London, with twenty-two years in the Greenwich branch of the London Mission. Like his father-in-law, he had a deeply evangelical faith, and an awareness that the gospel, to be meaningful, must be translated into terms of compassion and service. Then, in 1940, he was set free from circuit work to become the secretary of the Trust.

It was in no way surprising, then, that Hilda Bartlett Lang had a great fund of compassion. Nor was it unexpected that, in the early days of the war, she should respond to Walter Hall's idea of a home for the aged—though where and how she heard of it is something she has quite forgotten. In the early 1940s she had taken the family to live in Plymouth, her husband's home town.

Then, after the Plymouth blitz, they moved to Bognor Regis, on the south coast. It was here that she began to collect for a home for the elderly—and she had Bognor itself in mind. *That* home, however, was not to appear on the MHA lists for some time to come. But even in Bognor the war was not far away. As she cycled home one night in the black-out, Mrs Lang heard the crash of a bomb and immediately afterwards found herself on the ground with the cycle on top of her.

It was from Bognor that Mrs Lang wrote to Walter Hall, then at Conference in Leeds, making the offer on behalf of the Rank Trust that was to assure the approval of the Conference for the Homes themselves and for the Capital Fund appeal of £60,000. By that time her own association with the MHA was well defined as its treasurer, and in the years to come Walter Hall, living at Selsdon with his wife, was to become a close and valued friend when the Langs moved to Reigate after the war.

One of the best-known journalists in Methodism was H. L. Gee, a Yorkshireman who turned out a long and swift succession of best-selling books and was known to readers of a popular newspaper as 'Francis Gay'. Though his essays, in which he described himself as striding across the moors, pictured a large and vigorous character, he was in fact short and slight. But there was nothing small about his generous spirit. Another Methodist literary figure was Sydney Walton, who gave his creations in *Who's Who* as writing, reading and talking. The first widely distributed piece of publicity on behalf of the new Methodist Homes for the Aged was the work of these two writers.

It was a four-page broadsheet, dated 'Summertime 1945' and entitled *The Evening Chair*. Few copies have survived, and it has been impossible to trace a copy of the booklet which Sydney Walton agreed to write about the early struggles to establish the Homes. Sentimental in approach, it was typical of both writers, but considering their wide readership it would seem to have been assured of a general appeal. There is, however, no indication of how widespread its circulation in Methodism may have been. It nevertheless includes a good deal of information which shows how far the organization had moved in its first few months of existence.

Sydney Walton had a fulsome paragraph. 'To keep the faith right into old age, to hold the joy of faith while the sun is setting, to hold youth in the heart though flesh be feeble; that is grandeur and it is to those amongst our Methodist folk that we wish to express our praise and thanksgiving in the form of homes of affection in which the evening chair is honoured and exalted.' Lush prose of that kind has no place in modern MHA publicity, but there is another respect in which the broadsheet has a 'period' flavour.

It has one single picture—an aged lady in an 'evening chair', her black satin dress covering all but the toes of her shoes, a cameo brooch holding her black shawl and a very obvious hairnet gripping her white hair. 'Light at evening time, and a hearth for the feet', says the caption. There are few of today's residents, even the oldest, who would see themselves reflected in such a picture. Not only do they have no hearths; they are much more smartly dressed.

But the picture no doubt typifies how people of the war years imagined age at its best—tidy, rather feeble, out of touch with the world. Walton's appeal had the same pre-war patina. '£60,000 seems trivial by the side of our compassions. If we break up the total into little sums, into sixpences and shillings and ten-shilling notes and pound notes, and resolve each of us to contribute our moiety, the treasury soon will overflow.'

We may now sniff slightingly about the style of the writing, but the message was plain. The success or failure of the homes in those earliest days would depend on small gifts by the hundred from people who could never afford large ones. And, over the next few years, they came—a generous, touching stream from all over the country, and many of them from people who were elderly themselves.

There were more significant references—to Wallington, Tankerton and Harrogate. There was a paragraph about the 'Flower Fund' and a mention of Margaret Harwood. All the names indicated a burgeoning interest. But perhaps the most revealing article is an interview with Walter Hall, in H. L. Gee's inimitable style. He quotes directly from Hall's own words.

'While the war lasts and building materials are restricted, we do not propose building homes ourselves. There are many large houses in country districts which are both available and cheap, but most of them are not very suitable for the needs of the aged. They are too isolated from churches and congenial Christian fellowship, and from what I may call the main stream of life. Further, though the aged are our immediate objective, we hope and intend ultimately *to provide accommodation for supernumerary ministers and their wives, retired missionaries, Sisters, and NCHO workers and local preachers.*'

That was a far cry from the limited objectives Hall had put before the Conference, and they were never to be achieved. But Methodism itself, stimulated by others who shared Hall's concerns, was to undertake—for local preachers and retired ministers, for instance—some of the things the MHA was never large enough or qualified to do.

One of his main points, however—the necessity for homes to be within 'the main stream of life'—was to become a fundamental criterion for those who planned the homes.

Despite the comparatively small amount of publicity a good many Methodists quickly heard about the homes. An increasing number of Hall's letters contained appeals for help, many of them pathetic.

'I live in a bed-sitting room. I am not complaining, but there is always the thought of the loneliness of the near future. I am quite alone in the world.'

A daughter wrote about her father. 'I do beg of you to consider his application. Another winter alone frightens him.'

A woman of seventy-five wrote of the difficulty of finding accommodation. 'I am weary tramping about to find somewhere to stay. It would be grand not to worry any more.'

To meet such a stream of appeals immediately would be impossible. But even before Hall had his final go-ahead from the Conference a beginning had been made.

In the summer of 1943 committee members began the search for properties in both north and south. Hall asked Mrs Middlemiss and Mrs J. K. Whitehead to join Mrs Lang in seeking somewhere suitable. 'There was some man, too', Mrs Lang recalled years later, and dismissed him in a phrase. 'He wasn't much use, though!' A house in Streatham Park seemed possible at first, but unsatisfactory on inspection. It was the same with others. Then a committee member, Mr Cropper, reported that a house in Beddington Gardens at Wallington, in Surrey, was in the market for £3,000—but the owner would take £2,700 if it were to be used for an old people's home. Adapting it would cost perhaps £500. There was not that much in the funds, but the Midland Bank—the traditional bank of the Methodist Church—might be prepared to arrange an overdraft of £4,000.

On 6th January 1944—a historic day—it was agreed to complete the purchase of Ryelands, the Wallington house.

But who would decide on the applicants? That January meeting was left in no doubt that there would be far more than enough for Ryelands.

'We have already had sixty-five applications', announced Walter Hall.

By the annual committee meeting in May 1944, the number had risen to 130. They included, amongst others, twenty-eight widows, thirty-five spinsters, six widowers, four deaconesses, fifteen local preachers or their relatives, and twenty ministers or relatives of ministers. It was a formidable list and clearly exposed only a tiny part of the hidden mass of needy people.

Sister Frances Topping was appointed the first matron of this first home—on a trial period of six months, at a salary of £1 a week.

It was finally agreed that applications from widows and spinsters aged not more than seventy-five would be considered—that cut out a considerable number of applications both on the grounds of age and sex—and that no final decision would be reached until a formal questionnaire had been answered. This became the normal procedure of the MHA in its early days.

In H. L. Gee's broadsheet Hall also stressed a number of practical points.

Offers of service had been accepted from women who desired to devote their lives to the service of the aged through the MHA.

Other offers of service would be welcomed.

Most residents wished to furnish their own rooms, but additional furnishings would be required, such as rugs and carpets, articles for the dining-room and the lounge. Those who had surplus linen, curtain material or furniture were urged to provide them, on the understanding that what was not suitable might be 'disposed of' for the general fund of the Homes, though prospective donors were wisely asked to send to Hall himself a description of what they were prepared to offer.

He was able, too, to indicate that cash was beginning to arrive. Offers of money in memory of parents or friends, and intimation of wills made in favour of the Homes, were encouraging. Under enthusiastic leadership one circuit had contributed £77—a large amount in 1945. Women's Fellowships and Sisterhoods were already expressing an interest, and much more might be done through these organizations.

One important long-term element in the budget of the Home had already come into existence. Sydney Walton, in *The Evening Chair*, drew attention to 'a suggestion that first grew amongst the Scandinavian snows and which took root and spread in Harrow (his home town) during the war'. Instead of putting flowers on graves, Harrow residents made 'gifts of money to the Hospital on the Hill, gifts which were translated into living ministries of healing'. Why should not the same be done for the Methodist Homes for the Aged. Mrs Middlemiss, of North London (he reported) had already taken up the idea. She had called it the 'Flower Fund' and a small printed leaflet was in circulation. 'Margaret Harwood of the human pen'—Walton's own description—had drawn it to the attention of her many readers in the *Methodist Recorder*.

By the summer of 1945 gifts for the Flower Fund totalled £773—and, of this, £554 had come through Margaret Harwood.

This pseudonym of the Isle of Wight journalist, Sybil Haddock, was to be linked closely with MHA for the next thirty years, and she was to bring in a very large sum for the MHA during that time, especially through her Christmas appeal.

The Flower Fund, from its small beginning, has grown enormously through the years. The 1945 total of £773 had increased to £2,500 by 1960, and in 1970 it brought in £5,899. Two years later it was over £9,000 and by 1975 had reached £11,500.

Between the Conference of 1943 which had given 'general approval' to Walter Hall's proposals and the 1944 Conference which formally established the Methodist Homes for the Aged, the first house had been bought at Wallington and its first matron appointed. Before the summer of 1945 some applicants had been accepted and had taken up residence. Walter Hall himself was busier than ever. He was a man of rare ability, idealism and courage. Intending to retire in the summer of 1940, the pressures of war had made him agree to continue as chairman of the London North District, one of the greatly devasted areas of Methodism. He was still minister of the church at Tottenham. Now, in addition, he had the responsibility of this new and growing organization. Methodist ministers did not have secretaries in those days, and for Walter Hall his office was his own home. The headquarters of the Methodist Homes for the Aged was his study at Firgrove, in the little Surrey town of Selsdon.

5

The Chairman

Harrogate

Privacy, a real community life, one's own personal possessions—in short, the possibility of 'one's own home within a home'—was an almost entirely new concept in care for the aged. Enthusiasm, doggedness, compassion and administrative skills were essential qualities in one who was to prove that such an idea was realistic. Walter Hall possessed them to the full, as well as being well known and respected amongst those who knew the official life and personalities of Methodism. But this was not enough to ensure the more general response that would quickly be needed.

Such a venture really demanded strong lay support, the advocacy and acumen of a man engaged in commerce or industry, influential with local authorities or government ministries, a person of consequence outside Methodism as well as within it. If such a man were not only a person of character but a 'character' in himself, and if he could be found in the north rather than the south where supporters already existed, the advantage of such additional leadership would be enormous.

Hall had not far to seek for such a man. All these qualifications were, in fact, to be found in the vigorous, competitive and wealthy chairman of the new committee. Sir George Martin was already one of the best-known figures in the North of England, a man with a caring heart who would ensure a proper amalgam of shrewdness and compassion in the committee's approach to its work. It was to be said of him when he relinquished the chairmanship thirty years later that he had 'insisted on the highest standards . . . built with the future in mind . . . allowed no slapdash solution to any problem to pass his examination . . . and that the financial position of the 1970s owed much to his genius'.

George William Martin had Methodism in his blood and bones, and the strength of his loyalty to it was reinforced by the family tradition of his wife. His father was a Methodist minister, Edward Martin; his grandfather on his mother's side, Dr George Osborn, one of Wesleyan Methodism's greatest Missionary Secretaries, had twice been president of the Methodist Conference. George Martin was born in South Norwood, in London, 1884, one of a family of seven, though his life-long associations have been with Yorkshire and especially with Leeds. His brothers and sisters, like the children of many manses, were to find their future in professional circles. One sister was a teacher and two others were closely linked with the life of Methodism through their husbands, for one was a minister and the other a medical missionary in India.

George himself, however, went into commerce. It was not his first choice. He really wanted to be a farmer but his father brushed off such folly. 'You need too much capital', he said, 'and *I* haven't got any! Wait till you're older and have got some of your own.' In the end, George Martin *did* find a farm, at Copgrove, five miles from Harrogate, but that was when he was almost seventy and able to enjoy what some people (not knowing of his early hopes) regarded as an elderly whim—out of the fortune he had made in commerce. He has a prize herd of Jersey cattle and in his dining-room are six silver cups, one of them for the Supreme Champion. He still visits the farm on Sunday—and it would be unlike him not to breed champions!

Before he retired as chairman he was to add to his great generosity by giving the valuable Scruton Grange Farm, then valued at £72,000, to the MHA as one of its major assets.

In fact, he began his commercial career in the office of a firm which manufactured raincoats, but he soon moved to another position. This was with Wilkinson, Warburton Ltd., a firm of wholesale dealers in domestic goods, furnishings, clothing and a wide range of related products. It was to become, in time, a large and highly profitable undertaking, providing a fortune for the young man who, on his appointment, chose to reject an attractive annual salary in favour of a lower one of his own choosing with a commission attached to it. Though he had only a small margin at the end of the first year, he *was* on the right side, and he very quickly proved his value to the firm, making his way swiftly until he became a partner. The unexpected deaths of senior partners gave him important responsibility very early in life and he began to transform the firm into a modern, competitive business with large outlets and a broad sweep of business. For many years he has been chairman of the board of directors.

MHA has benefited directly from his association with Wilkinson, Warburton Ltd, since it provided furnishings for the homes in Cramlington, Hitchin, Hull, Lincoln and Scarborough.

He had a good many other interests, besides his repressed love of farming. His recreation is listed as 'shooting' in *Who's Who*, which devotes nearly a whole column to his activities and achievements.

Always fond of music, with a good singing voice, he became closely associated with the musical life of Leeds, his home city. From 1942–54 he was chairman of the Leeds Musical Festival. Sir Thomas Beecham and Sir Malcolm Sargent were amongst his friends, and guests at Adel Lodge, his solid and impressive, though not opulent, home a few miles from the city centre.

He was knighted in 1935, at the age of fifty, when he was made a K.B.E. It was an honour which he had already earned through his involvement in municipal life, but that period only marked the real beginning of much greater influence in municipal, county and national affairs. More distinctive than his knighthood was his appointment in 1954 as High Sheriff of Yorkshire, a rare honour indeed, and he is also the only surviving Honorary Freeman of the City of Leeds, with which dignity he was invested in 1966.

He had a great interest in the University of Leeds, of which he was a generous benefactor, and was for ten years a member of its Council and Court. Nearer to Bradford is the Methodist public school, Woodhouse Grove, and here too he was open-handed in his support. From about the end of the war to the 1970s he was chairman of the Board of Governors, and still remains a governor.

Perhaps the deepest commitment of his life, however, has been to hospital affairs and public health, and, through this concern, to the needs of the aged. In a more general but associated field he was closely concerned in the setting up of the National Health Service. It was in the 1920s that he became involved in local government and, since every member of a municipality must take his share of committee work, found himself engaged in the National Assistance and Health Committees of the city of Leeds. His interest was quickly captured. Few items escaped his notice in business affairs and the same was true of his committee work. Hospital wards in those days bore little resemblance to present-day standards, and many of the indigent aged were housed in the workhouses. George Martin was horrified at the crowded conditions, the almost complete lack of decent amenities and the unnecessary suffering of the patients. He decided to find out the worst—and discovered that it was far worse than he had imagined.

One visit was to remain ineradicably in his mind and to condition the direction of his activities. It was to a typical workhouse. At the entrance to one ward with Harold Fieldhouse, the executive officer of the committee, he stopped short and pulled out his handkerchief to cover his mouth. When he took it away the fetid odour clung to him. The stench of the ward was unbearable.

'Who are these old men?' he demanded.

The ward nurse was polite, but impatient with visiting committee members. 'Cancer cases . . . things like that . . . they're all incurable . . . or else just senile. You can't do anything for them; that's why they're here. They're waiting to die.'

Those thirty-six old men, crowded close together in a ward with wooden floorboards stained by half a century of dirt and ordure, its windows high in the peeling walls letting out little of the nauseating smell, were to be the memory which would, for Sir George Martin, symbolize the most repellent aspects of 'care' for the aged. He was not alone in his horrified response to such scenes, nor was he the only one to determine to change things. More people than he realized had heard the anguish which had caught at Walter Hall's heart—'Don't let me go to the Union!' George Martin could understand for the first time why the poor had this inescapable dread.

'This must be changed', he said angrily to his colleague, Fieldhouse.

Most of the 1940s were to pass before the workhouse system began to give way to more humane conditions. Meanwhile, Martin and Fieldhouse began their own private campaign. In the

1920s and '30s, with the new equalities brought about by World War I, old-type servants were becoming scarcer, and those who had worked for better wages in factories were not content to see their children 'go into service', with the long hours, the little money and the snobbery which such work incurred. Even wealthy Yorkshire millers and businessmen were finding it difficult to maintain their large establishments, and their houses were coming on to the market as they exchanged them for less pretentious ones.

Martin and Fieldhouse, with the backing of their committees, began buying some of these houses and turning them into 'homes' for old people. Each home had space for thirty or forty elderly people, housed in dormitories with half a dozen beds instead of the slummy conditions of the workhouse. There was a common-room for those who were mobile, and nursing for those who were bed-ridden. It was a long and courageous step along the road towards the rehabilitation of 'care for the elderly'. As it turned out, it was also to be important in the development of the then-unconceived Methodist Homes for the Aged. It meant that when Hall, in the early 1940s, began to seek out those who shared his enthusiasm he was able to find a tough, sometimes ruthless, realistic Methodist layman of distinction in Yorkshire who already had experience of the very thing he himself was planning.

It was the minister of Martin's own church, Lorne Cornish, who set things moving. Cornish, who was associated with the Methodist headquarters at Westminster, came to see him one day.

'Sir George, we want your help. A friend of mine, Walter Hall, is anxious to do something to help old people in Methodism who can't find homes to live in. You've got some experience of this sort of thing. Will you give him the benefit of your advice when you're next in London?'

In fact, Martin attended the first mid-war committee—an informal gathering of half a dozen people who met to hear Hall expound his hopes. 'It's a problem that's going to increase', he urged. 'People are living five or ten years longer than they used to do. It's no use putting things off.'

'Not even until the war is over?' questioned one of them. 'It's a bad time to start something now . . . everyone thinking of their own future . . . putting all they've got into the war effort . . . buildings being bombed everywhere!'

That was not a philosophy which appealed to Sir George Martin. 'Things never get easier by leaving them till later. I think we should act—and act at once. We should go to the Conference and ask for their approval'

It was that meeting which led to Hall's first appeal to the Conference in 1942. The informal group became a committee. More quickly than even the most optimistic had believed likely the Methodist Homes for the Aged were constituted and Sir George Martin, K.B.E., LL.D., was appointed its vigorous and far-sighted chairman.

Still alert and knowledgeable, though now over ninety, he remains in the grey-stone house where he has lived for more than fifty years, though much of the joy went out of life when his wife died. The same elderly man comes in each week, moving quietly through the big, crowded rooms to wind up the clocks. The limousine draws round to the door to take him to his office and warehouse in Pudsey almost every day, or to the club for a meal at noon. Ask him what has given him the greatest satisfaction in life and it will not be work, much as he has enjoyed it, or his money, though that has enabled him to be extremely generous. It is more likely to be his interest in health affairs—he was for many years the chairman and treasurer of the Yorkshire Council for Cancer Research—and hospital development. (It was a well-deserved tribute when the Leeds General Infirmany honoured him by naming a new five-storey block the 'Martin Wing', which was opened by H.R.H. the Duke of Edinburgh.) Close behind has been his dedicated interest in the Methodist Homes for the Aged. What he has meant to that organization is beyond computation.

Once the MHA was set up, appeals for help began to arrive by almost every post.

'The rooms are needed and we must look out for another place.'

'I have to find a new home and have been to eighteen places

this week, but all to no avail. No one will take permanent guests now—only holiday folk paying high prices.'

Walter Hall shared the letters with Sir George and his treasurer, Mrs Lang—who had her eye on Bognor as a possible site. She was still living there and the 'mulberry harbour' was being constructed just outside for the invasion of Normandy and Europe. But the Canadian army was in possession of a house she coveted. Sir George, too, was beginning to keep his eyes open for possibilities in the north.

It was when he was playing bridge at his club with a solicitor friend that he remarked how miserable he looked.

'You'd be unhappy, too, George. It's all right for you, with Adel Lodge and people to run it. I had to give up Berwick Grange in Harrogate because I couldn't keep it going.'

'I thought some London firm was using it as their head office?'

'They were. But they don't find Harrogate easy. They're giving it up and going back to London. I shall have to try to sell it—but who wants to buy a house like that now?'

Sir George kept the gleam out of his eye. 'How much do you want for it?'

'£6,000.'

The conversation moved back to the bridge hands. But that night Sir George drove from his Leeds home to Harrogate in the black-out. He parked his car quietly, took his torch and pushed open the gate at Berwick Grange. By torch-light, discreetly shrouded, he examined the house. An early Victorian mansion, of the typical mill-owner style, it had a wonderful garden and a useful gardener's cottage. He wandered round it all, stumbled here and there, and drove home.

Next day, back at the club, he chose to eat lunch with his friend. 'That house of yours—I'll give you £5,000 for it.'

The solicitor was startled, but his Yorkshire business sense masked his desire to sell. 'I'd rather let the estate agents have it. They'd get more.'

'If you do you'll only lose £500 in expenses. I'll split the difference—and give you £5,500!'

'Very well, I'll take it.'

In St Peter's church, in Leeds, is the gravestone of John Wesley's first woman preacher, Sarah Crosby. This part of Yorkshire has associations with Methodism reaching back to the days of its founder. Harrogate, a spa town, has strong Methodist churches, and was widely known and much visited by north-country people. Especially after the war, it was a favourite place for holiday-makers, tourists and conferences. Ripon and Knaresborough, both famous sight-seeing places, are not far away; nor is Harewood House. But Harrogate's great glory is the Stray, a magnificent lawn-like, tree-studded common of more than 200 acres, stretching crescent-like round the centre of the town. Berwick Grange faces directly on to this lovely open land.

There are several problems implicit in writing about the Methodist Homes for the Aged. One is that such a book might well deteriorate into a dull, reiterative description of more than thirty buildings which, however different in some ways, essentially consist of small residential rooms, large communal rooms, staff quarters and domestic areas. Nothing, after a few such accounts, could be more tedious—except for the staff and residents in the place being described! A second difficulty is that to spotlight one or two residents or staff members is to leave out others—so, even where such people are picked out here and there, they will remain anonymous. In any case, the few only illustrate the character, courage, initiative and individuality of something more than 1,000 residents or the devoted and loving service of more than 300 members of staff.

A third hurdle to be overcome is that to describe, first, each home at the time it came into the MHA lists and then attempt to outline the subsequent alterations and extensions that have taken place, would be confusing and awkward. In general, then, where a home is described at any length it will be as the visitor would find it today. So then to Harrogate.

Solid, quietly opulent as was proper for a wealthy, Yorkshire businessman's home, and built of grey stone, it has a settled, comfortable aspect which hardly prepares one for the splendour of the square hall. Here a fine staircase rises, its single flight dividing half-way up and turning back and upwards. Beautiful iron balustrades give a light touch, and the magnificent stained-glass window behind the stairs, reaching to the roof, provides an element of richness. Wedgwood and white walls in the hall, and a ceiling with ornamental plaster-reliefs and deep red and blue bosses, add their own touches to the grandeur.

Such an entry into magnificence is deceptive. It might well be over-powering to elderly people from very different surroundings, for the same sense of dignity is found throughout the house. But the residents, enjoying it all, are far from overwhelmed. Living in their own rooms, which vary in size, they remain completely themselves.

As well as anywhere, Berwick Grange shows the pattern of all the homes. Each resident has his or her own room, though some accommodate husband and wife. That they bring their own furniture is part of the special genius behind the life of the homes. (Only rooms in the 'special' homes for those needing additional care and attention are furnished, by the MHA.) They can use their rooms as much or as little as they like; have friends to visit them when they wish; sit up, lie down, rest or fill in their time according to their own inclinations without any sense of being supervised, ordered or pried upon.

Their rooms are their own homes, transferred into a larger community of the kind they have known and grown up with.

Berwick Grange has a very large lounge, with attractive views of the lovely gardens. There is a TV room—in almost every home this is separate from the main lounge—and a dining-room with tables accommodating small groups. In some homes there are tables for three, or for half a dozen; in most cases they are laid for four. They show no institutional laminated tops, clattering to crockery and cutlery, but clean and attractive tablecloths.

The staff, too, is fairly typical, though it varies in numbers from place to place, usually because of unfilled gaps.

Probably the most urgent need of the MHA at any time of the year is for more staff, and especially for residential staff

A resident matron is a 'must'. So is an assistant matron, though there are too many gaps in this category. Both matron and assistant must love elderly people and find pleasure in their work. They need an ability to care without fussing, to guide without ordering, to listen without seeming to do so with only one ear, to be as caring and patient with staff as with residents, and to cope with the unexpected. They will never be bored by monotonous routine!

Whenever one is obtainable there should be a resident cook and, in addition, two or three other resident helpers, as well as a number of non-resident workers. Berwick Grange, in holiday-time, provided an interesting mixture of 'stand-in' workers—three students, including senior schoolgirls, all bright and happy in their temporary work, and an acting cook who was a third-year trainee-teacher specializing in French. The cuisine was as British as the residents could have wished!

'What do the residents do with their time, when they're not sitting in their rooms?' The inevitable question will always produce some interesting answers.

'We can potter in the garden if we want to . . . some of us do an extra bit of washing for any men who can't do it for themselves . . . and some ironing and mending for them, too, if they're a bit helpless!'

'Of course we can always go out if we want to. We're very near the shops—and the church is really just at the back of the house.'

One elderly lady, in her eighties, is watching the test match on TV. 'Are you interested in cricket?' The reply is predictable from a Yorkshire-woman, though not the comment from another resident.

'She fell down and broke her wrist when she was at cricket. She got excited, I think. Her friends took her to hospital to get it set. She wouldn't let them stay, though . . . made them go back to watch the end of the match. After all, they'd paid for it!'

At Berwick Grange the twenty-four residents were mainly over eighty, and some of the most vigorous over ninety. That, like most of the other things in this Harrogate home, is typical of any the homes you may visit.

Next door to Berwick Grange is a second house belonging to the MHA, offering accommodation to retired workers in the Homes. But that is another, and much later, development in the story.

6

The problems of peace

Tankerton/Ilkley/Liverpool/Bognor/Hathersage

The third house opened by the Methodist Homes for the Aged was welcoming its first residents within two years of the organization's official beginning.

To reach the east coast of Kent, or the mouth of the Thames estuary, from London the journey moves from suburban towns to the cathedral city of Rochester, on through fruit orchards and hop-gardens with their conical oast-houses, out past flat marshlands where thousands of sheep nibble amongst the rushes, to seaside towns of no special beauty like Whitstable and Herne Bay. It was here than an estate agent suggested that the MHA should look at 'a very desirable property'. It was a small hotel, facing out to sea, at Tankerton—a town which has grown up alongside Whitstable. Whitstable itself has been famous for little other than the oysters which have been eaten and prized here since the days of Julius Caesar. It has a Methodist church built during the ministry of Richard Connell, the grandfather of the third ministerial secretary of the MHA.

No one would claim that Cliff Dene, on Marine Drive at Tankerton, was MHA's 'best buy'. Today, with some twenty-four residents, there is no room for expansion in any direction except on the roof, and very little room there! Residents' rooms are average in size, but the public rooms are not. From the staff point of view there is little elbow-room, and the garden is tiny.

But when Tankerton was bought it must have seemed very well suited to its purpose. There was a home in the south and another in the north; it was perhaps right to have another in the south-east. It has the advantages of being near to shops, sea and local churches—and the need of such amenities being accessible to elderly people was something which the committee took to heart very quickly. With its first half-dozen residents, and then its first dozen, there was plenty of room for everybody—and that was as far as the committee could go, with a very limited choice of housing at prices they could pay. At that stage, despite Harrogate, they were unable to plan for days when thirty would be an economic number of residents. Wallington, the first home, had less than a dozen and Berwick Grange, which in any case, had been enlarged, were the result of shrewd bargaining.

The MHA committee was to learn a good deal from the positive advantages—good fresh air and accessibility to amenities amongst them—and the disadvantages of such homes as Tankerton and, a little later, Liverpool. Not everybody, of course, appreciated the fresh air. A Cornish-woman who was one of the original residents at Tankerton thought of applying for a transfer to Cornwall many years later when the Falmouth home was opened.

'These cold-east winds are killing me!' she complained.

But she still lived on to be ninety-eight—and died at Tankerton. To permit transfers from one home to another would, in any case, be impracticable for a wide variety of good reasons, and is not allowed.

In the early days of the organization, as throughout its history, the 'right' sort of staff was a matter of supreme importance. The women who became the first residential staff were chosen partly because of their capability and character, and partly because they were felt by the committee to have a due sense of vocation. But there have always been hazards in this matter of vocation. By a century-old tradition in British life, going back to the days of Florence Nightingale, the appeal for vocational service had been made to 'ladies of means' who would find adequate fulfilment in 'vocation' since they needed little extra money to live on. As the intake of the nursing service broadened to accept applicants from a much wider social spectrum, it was assumed that the same high-minded idealism prevailed—the pleasure of doing things for others ought to outweigh the disadvantages of little money and inadequate accommodation. The MHA was not free of this attitude.

In recent years the MHA has taken long strides forward in terms both of pay and accommodation. It has had to do so to keep pace with other statutory welfare professions. Even so, a major preoccupation in the immediate future must be with staff accommodation in the older homes—no easy matter, in some cases, because such houses are not readily adaptable. For far too long the welfare services suffered from the unworldly idea that 'service' was almost enough in itself. The MHA was peculiarly fortunate that most of those who joined its ranks did, in fact, rate service very highly indeed. For them, social obligation to the needy was matched with a sense of Christian joy.

Walter Hall had originally intended to retire in 1940. The war prevented it and he was still in harness when the war ended in 1945. That year he retired from the active work of the ministry. But he still continued his work as the secretary of the MHA. Already things had moved a long way from one of his early appeals when he wrote that because there were no homes in British Methodism he knew of women who were applying for entrance to John Wesley's original 'Home for Widows' in Dublin! Methodism had not only begun to catch up, but it was moving fast.

One of the deep-rooted, city rivalries in Britain has been that between Leeds and Bradford. The same friendly rivalry existed between the Leeds and Bradford Methodist Districts. Soon after the completion of the purchase of Berwick Lodge Sir George Martin went to church, as he normally did, at Headingley. The preacher was a very distinguished minister, Dr Russell Maltby. Sir George did not listen very intently to the sermon. He was thinking about Leeds . . . and Bradford . . . and hatching a private plan. Dr Maltby was Warden of the Deaconess Institute at Ilkley—and Ilkley was to Bradford what Harrogate was to Leeds, both in social and Methodist terms.

When the service ended he went into the vestry to talk to his friend about the splendid Berwick Grange in Harrogate.

'Don't you think Bradford needs a home like this, too, Maltby?'

The question was enough. On the Wednesday morning he had a phone call from Dr Maltby. 'I think I've found just what we want. A house called Glen Rosa.'

'Where's that?'

'At Ilkley.' Just where Dr Malby lived; not far from the Deaconess Institute itself. If the Leeds district were anxious to make Berwick Grange a fine home, Bradford would need no stimulus to do the same at Ilkley. 'It's a lovely house . . . two lodges . . . over an acre of fine gardens. And we could get it for £8,500,' Maltby ended.

Sir George was at Ilkley as fast as his car could take him.

Glen Rosa was opened to its first residents in 1947.

It is undoubtedly a lovely home—though whether it is better than Berwick Grange depends on whether you ask the residents in Ilkley or Harrogate! Grey stone; dignity; beautifully kept lawns and flower-gardens shaded by lovely trees; magnificent views over wooded hills towards the dales, with the moors in sight; a wide residential road but no traffic noise; space to sit out in the sun . . . all these make for the comfort and peace of the residents. Everywhere there is an air of grace.

Today a new wing for more residents, excellent additions to the kitchen, a lift (Glen Rosa was the only home without one), and a new staff sitting-room have been added to the public rooms and residential accommodation which were built when the house was taken over.

Had Sir George Martin's contribution to the MHA been only the provision of Berwick Grange and Glen Rosa it would have been very considerable indeed.

Peace came at last, in August 1945, when Japan capitulated after the horror of the atomic explosion at Hiroshima. To say that it was a different world from that of the 1930s is, of course, the grossest understatement. Attitudes, hopes, standards and ideals had altered as much as the shattered aspect of Britain's bombed cities. Perhaps the most significant change came with the general election of 1945. Winston Churchill lost his seat in parliament, to the incredulous astonishment of Britain's allies, and a Labour government came to power in a landslide victory. They brought a commitment to a new style of life—the continued acceptance of austerity with the promise of a Welfare State in which no one would ever again suffer the degradations that many workers had known in the 1930s and a host of older people throughout their lives.

The basis of the new concept of the Welfare State and the legislation which would create it was the 'Beveridge Plan', the work of a committee but signed by Sir William Beveridge alone, which had been published in 1942. It was designed to offer security to many who were without rights, or who had minimal assistance from the state. Amongst these were the aged, and especially the poor.

There were other signs of a changing world. Coal was nationalised in 1946, followed quickly by electricity, iron and steel. India gained independence, the separate nation of Pakistan was born—and true-blue Tory faces grew red with indignation as 'the Socialists began to give away the British Empire'. The school-leaving age was raised to fifteen. Britain suffered the worst snow conditions for sixty years and—adding a little human gaiety to a still-drab scene—Princess Elizabeth and Prince Philip were married in Westminster Abbey.

In Liverpool the docks were again getting busy with normal traffic instead of troopships, the Mersey tunnel was still comparatively uncongested because of petrol rationing, and no one had thought of restoring the magnificent Victorian gothic public buildings from their black grime to their original stone colour. Tommy Handley was only one of the unending stream of comedians to come out of Liverpool, but for years he had brought spontaneous merriment to an embattled nation with ITMA.

Not far from Tommy Handley's old home at Aigburth, in South Liverpool, were several well-preserved green 'lungs' of the city. There was Otterspool Park, which had once had a zoo, between the main road to Widnes and the river Mersey. Near by was Sefton Park, much bigger, ringed with great houses built by merchants who had inherited fortunes made from slavery. And by Otterspool Park, running from the main road to the river, was Fulwood Park—'millionaire's row'—with houses as arrogant as any in the city.

'Yer got to take yer boots off to walk down there', jeered the local boys.

But, in any case, 'getting down there' had not been easy. There had been a lodge at the entrance to Fulwood Park, with a gate spanning the road and a gatekeeper to open it for carriages and, later, for cars. Now, like much else, Fulwood Park was changing too. In time the big houses would become flats, nurseries or child-care centres. For the moment, the problem was how to get rid of houses of that size. As in Harrogate and Ilkley, stately homes were impossible to staff and expensive to maintain.

One of them, number 19, was owned by Mr Cohen, founder of Lewis's, Liverpool's most patronized popular store, and it was this house, with its pillared verandah and its large window lighting the billiard-room, which was purchased by the MHA. It was opened in 1948. Bigger than Tankerton, more austere than Harrogate or Ilkley, its major disadvantage was its distance from the main road and shops. A second disability was a basement kitchen (its removal to the ground floor is only comparatively recent). To the Rev. George H. Taylor, a founder-member of the MHA committee, the difficulties may have been evident, but they were outweighed by the desirability of having the fifth MHA homes sited in Merseyside, in the busy north-west of the country.

At the back of the house is a not over-large garden with pleasant lawns—an ideal place for the annual summer sale organized by the residents and the ladies' committee.

These 'local' committees vary. In some places they are very active; in one or two places they do not exist effectively at all. Composed of women from churches in the area—and, in this case, from the 'over the water' too—they may visit the home from time to time; help to organize coffee mornings or annual sales, and bring friends to buy at them; stimulate interest in their own churches and circuits. Liverpool and Harrogate exemplify places where their support for the matron has been personal and their service to the residents has made for the smooth running of the home at times when it was under pressure. They have 'stood in' when there was a shortage of staff, or at weekends, looking after the tea or working in the kitchen. They have 'taken over' when the staff have gone out together for a rare 'evening off'. Such local committees, are more likely to be a valuable publicity agency for the work of the home and to support the staff than to compete with the matron in trying to 'run the home'.

At Fulwood Park you may see a film of 'a year in the life of our home' made by one of the residents and widely shown in the district, or listen to reminiscences of Liverpool as it was just after the turn of the century, or find a man playing classics at an evening entertainment. To be 'over ninety' is, for people like this, a challenge to overcome the limitations of age rather than to give way to them.

Four years after the first 'challenge offer' from the Joseph Rank Benevolent Trust came a second. The £45,000 asked for in 1944 had been raised by support from within Methodism and the £15,000 paid over. This was no small achievement in the austere years round the ending of the war. Now came a second challenge —another £15,000; £1 for every £3 raised by the MHA.

If Mrs Lang's influence was itself a stimulus to the Trust it may well have been because of the possibilities now emerging at Bognor Regis.

Two of her friends, Miss Muddle and Miss Ballantyne, had joined her in seeking 'the right place' in the town where she and her family lived through most of the war. It was Mrs Lang who had made the discovery.

'It's in Hawthorn Road', she told Miss Ballantyne as they went to look at it. 'It's just what we're looking for. It used to be a boys' boarding school and now the Canadian army has it. When *they* get out *we* could get in.'

They examined it more closely when it came on the market. A charming, long, low house, its frontage given character by bay windows variously-constructed, its lower storey of brick and the upper one washed white with dormer windows above, it was full of character but without whimsy. Inside it was capacious, with rooms which could easily be turned into single bed-sittingrooms and pleasant lounges. There was a good vegetable garden and spacious lawns.

'They could use it for croquet', commented Miss Ballantyne. As, indeed, the residents now do.

On Whit Monday 1948, it was opened—appropriately by Mrs Lang herself, with her husband, the Rev. Fred Bartlett Lang, in the chair.

The local press reporter had a patronizing style, and a sense of the ridiculous might have encouraged him to use his blue pencil more freely. 'They have been hoping for fine weather so that they may enjoy outdoor jollifications . . . outside is a large shed which will be used for social and religious purposes.' Whether one resident really appreciated her press publicity may be doubted. 'I went into one room. A dresser—it might be thought old-fashioned—stands by a wall crowded with sepia reproductions in mahogany-coloured frames . . . an atmosphere of chintz with pot-pourri . . . the perfect setting for a little old lady.'

Little old ladies addicted to chintz and pot-pourri are now hard to find in the homes. Most of them are active, even if they are old; in many cases very active indeed. These Bognor residents have taken part in 'Age Concern' exhibitions in Chichester—and won prizes, amongst other entries, for tapestries that hang on their walls. They have knitted sixty blankets for Oxfam. They have an 'Easter bonnet parade' for the fun of it and, by contrast from four recent coffee mornings have given £100 to the Methodist Relief Fund and £100 to the Leprosy Mission as well as contributing to the purchase of a circuit minibus.

The reporter did get one thing right. He spoke of a room in which hung the portraits of two bewigged eighteenth-century clerical gentlemen. They were John and Charles Wesley, and the room's occupant was Mrs Edith Rhein, Charles Wesley's great-granddaughter. She had the aristocratic Wesley nose and, as Mrs Lang once remarked, 'although she was a dear she always knew what she wanted'.

It was Mrs Rhein's picture, seated and holding a picture of the great hymn-writer, which appeared on the second main piece of MHA publicity. This was a small booklet, *Good Evening*, which was written by the Rev. Fred Evison. Known to readers of the *Methodist Recorder* for a tongue-in-cheek children's column which was probably just as much read by adults and signed *F.H.E.*, Evison produced a better and more appealing brochure than *The Evening Chair*. The booklet included photographs of the seven homes then existing. By that time Wallington had eleven residents, Tankerton thirteen, Harrogate fourteen, Ilkley twelve. Liverpool and Bognor were larger, with thirty-one and twenty-four. The latest, with only half a dozen residents and only partly in occupation, was at Hathersage.

Hathersage is an attractive Derbyshire stone-built village, now greatly extended as a dormitory for Sheffield commuters. Set in the centre of the Derbyshire moors, it is within the magnificent Peak District and on the edge of the Peak National Park. Not far away are the Blue John mines and their near-by caves, and the beginning of the Pennine Way. In the churchyard lies Robin Hood's tall friend Little John. More people go to look at it than make pilgrimage to the house of the Eyre family, where Charlotte Brontë once worked and from where she took the name and setting for her most famous novel.

Just off the village square, facing across the moors, is Moorland House, the seventh home opened by the MHA. Its history is quite unlike any of the others.

When Walter Hall gained Conference approval for the setting up of the Methodist Homes he urged a number of practical suggestions. One was that districts or circuits might consider buying and opening their own homes. 'Don't leave it to the people in London to move first.' A fellow district chairman was William Wallace, of Sheffield. He had not forgotten Hall's appeal, and responded warmly to a letter from the Rev. Fred Stafford, an ex-army chaplain, who was then the superintendent minister of the Peak circuit. Could they not open a home for elderly people of the Sheffield district at Hathersage, asked Stafford.

Wallace was a fine preacher, a minister who had worked in central missions and knew the needs of his people, and a man of great compassion. But, though Stafford's idea appealed to him, he was too careful an administrator to build on emotion rather than practicalities. He went to see a Methodist bank manager, Seymour Bishop, who was the district treasurer for overseas missions and knew the financial capacities of the Sheffield people.

'Can we raise enough money to buy a home, equip it, and keep it going?'

'Certainly not just by a general appeal', counselled Bishop. 'It would mean a personal approach to people we think might help. I know a number of them.'

A committee was formed; the response to the appeal was generous. Two fairly large, square, stone-buillt houses, until recently occupied by a girls' school, were available in Hathersage. If they were purchased could the committee afford to run it?

'We don't want to come under London. It's better that we should do it ourselves. But we should ask them if they'd support us', suggested the treasurer.

The reply from London was clear. They would give what support they could from headquarters, but if Sheffield wanted a home in Hathersage they must buy it themselves. The six homes already in existence would tax the general resources for some time to come.

The Sheffield district, led by Wallace and Bishop, moved into action. They bought Moorland House and appealed for help—gifts for furnishing, money to buy essentials which would not be provided by the residents, women to scrub out, men to do running repairs and set the house in order. The help came, the sort of down-to-earth assistance expected in Derbyshire and Yorkshire. In 1949 Moorland House was opened to its first residents.

Between the original two houses there is now a two-storey connecting building, merging happily into the low, comfortable façade, and making a long attractive frontage above the slightly sloping lawn. No home is more accessible to church and shops, for the church is just round the corner and the square, crowded with tourists and walkers in the summer and quiet in the winter, is at the end of the road.

The residents take their share in contributing to the amenities of the home. In many rooms drawers and cardboard boxes are crowded with articles to be sold at the Open Day. There is the inevitable and essential embroidery in some boxes; the knitting in others. One room has a growing collection of professional-quality soft toys; another, a box of delightful finger-puppets. Few homes have more help from their residents in the sales they stage. The last Open Day here raised £550.

Other residents have other interests. Unforgettable is the minister who arrived with his telescope, well qualified to lecture on astronomy—but who thought that now he had time to spare, in his eighties, he would start to learn German. Another, a woman of eighty-five, an ex-teacher with several languages at her command, decided to learn Greek in order to read the New Testament in its original text—and stimulated a local doctor, without much church affiliation, to follow Paul's journeys on his summer holiday.

By the time Hathersage was opened Walter Hall had been able to retire. A new secretary, the Rev. William Stoate, was appointed by the Conference in his place in 1947. There were to be no dramatic changes in the immediate future—and indeed Stoate was to find the task of consolidation and development at least as hard as that which had faced Walter Hall at the beginning of the venture. But Hall, the true pioneer, was to live on until he was ninety, old, frail and blind, but keeping his interest in the homes, and his love of them, to the end of his life. Meanwhile, in the next decade, he was to remain active in the work of the committee, visiting possible sites, interviewing prospective staff and providing hope and encouragement to those who took over responsibility for the work he had begun.

The 1950s

Builders at work

'The Welfare State provides many things for old people, but it doesn't provide this—a warm and friendly welcome, good Christian fellowship with others of similar age and interests, and a combination of community life with a true respect for each other's privacy.'

—*Professor Charles A. Coulson*

7

The end of the Workhouse

Bath/Exmouth/Leamington

In the year 1952 King George VI died. The genuine grief of the British people, with whom he had shared the sufferings and privations of the war, was tempered by the enthusiasm which welcomed the new, young queen on her coronation. The ceremony was a boost to television sales and suddenly, for tens of thousands, TV became a fact of life. 'Come in, sit down, shut up, it's on' was to describe a new and frustrating style of domestic existence. Roger Bannister ran the first four-minute mile. Hilary and Sherpa Tensing climbed Everest. Sweet rationing ended in 1953, and *all* rationing the following year. Although the bank rate went up to 4½ per cent the 1950s heralded a bright, if not a brave, new world. But not for everyone; not, even in that decade, for the elderly.

In 1948 the Ministry of Health reported that 'the workhouse is doomed. Instead, local authorities are busy planning and opening small, comfortable homes where old people, many of them lonely, can live pleasantly and with dignity.' The statement, unhappily, was even less accurate than many government pronouncements.

A research writer on the care of the aged states that 'by the end of the war there were sufficient non-profit-making homes to provide a pattern for government development'. But he goes on to comment that government and local authorities were slow to learn from the pattern or to extend their own homes on the same model. Most voluntary homes were run by charitable or religious organizations. Some dated from the middle of the last century, and many of the oldest had been established to meet the needs of the poorest section of the population in the industrial cities. Some were adjuncts of older almshouses. There were 'retreats' for religious or professional people; quasi-hotels for the middle classes who could afford them. Many homes were run by Roman Catholic orders, a number by Jewish charities, a few, such as 'Homes for Lonely Christadelphians', belonged to minority groups. Methodists, in short, were by no means alone in this field of care for the elderly. In 1944 some 6,000 people were in homes run by twenty-six different religious bodies, and 3,000 in those maintained by other charities.

But several points need to be stressed about the homes that existed at this period. Two out of every five were in London, the home counties and Lancashire. Many were isolated, in large houses in the country; only half were anywhere near the edge of a city or town, and of the rest a large number were not even close to a village or a bus route. It was difficult for residents to 'get out' or for relatives and friends to visit, at a period when private transport was extremely limited. The majority had between thirty and forty beds; dormitories, or at least large shared bedrooms, were normal. Furnishings were provided by the organization.

The Nuffield Commission of 1947 had recommended that 'all normal old people who are no longer able to live an independent life should be accommodated in small homes rather than large institutions'. Such thinking undoubtedly spelt the death of crowded, unhygienic, inhuman workhouse conditions. But, even by 1960—thirteen years after the Nuffield report—too little progress had been made by local authorities. Even where local councils had a genuine sense of responsibility and caring the movement was slow. There was shortage of steel and money, a limitation on capital investment, an unwillingness in local communities, as distinct from municipal authorities, to take the problem seriously. Too few people regarded 'work amongst the old' as a worthwhile or financially rewarding occupation and, indeed, there was still a curious but widespread reluctance to accept *old* people as truly old *people*. The exceptions to these strictures glowed brightly but often in isolation, and the knowledgable and far-sighted Old People's Welfare Associations—much later to be summed up in 'Age Concern'—had to struggle hard against general inertia.

The Methodist contribution, small though it was, was of real significance. It was inspired by genuine care. Those who were accepted into the Methodist homes, even if they were not Methodists, quickly discovered a community of background, interest and even of acquaintance. Methodists have always had a strong sense of 'belonging to each other', and the 'connexional system' by which ministers moved widely throughout the country provided common links between many who entered the homes.

There were, however, some features of the Methodist Homes which were almost unique. First, the provision of individual bed-sitting-rooms with washbasins maintained a sense of privacy; second, the opportunity for residents to furnish their own rooms with their own belongings gave a secure feeling of being 'at home'; third, the careful but never grasping assessment of a resident's ability to pay was confidential—only the treasurer, never matron or staff, knew the amount paid. Each resident kept a feeling of personal dignity.

Other things also contribute to the characteristic style of life in these homes.

Rules are cut to a minimum. Residents live their own lives as they wish. They may go out when they want to; retire to their rooms when they wish; attend church meetings, clubs of one sort or another, or visit friends. There are no restrictions on visitors, no overhanging threat of 'having to ask matron'. Because of the lack of regimentation the atmosphere of 'being like home' is maintained and the proper dignity of age preserved.

'Old age' was clearly going to be an increasing, rather than a diminishing problem for state and community. Only statistics can illustrate the size of the problem.

In 1901 there were 1½ million people over sixty-five years of age; that was 5 per cent of the population. By 1911 the number had risen to 2 million; by 1939 to over 4 million—8 per cent of the population; by 1947 to 5 million; and by the 1950s to 6 million. By 1960 some 12 per cent of the population was over sixty-five years of age. In other words, between the time Walter Hall called together his first pre-war committee and the day when he handed over the secretaryship to William Stoate, there had been an addition of a million pensioners. By the time Stoate retired, ten years later, there was another million. Many of these were in the upper age-ranges, and they included an increasing number of frail people who could no longer look after themselves.

The MHA was created to care for those who could look after themselves, but what about the sick? The homes already opened could and do provide simple nursing of the sort offered within an ordinary family—but to run nursing homes was outside the capacity of the committee and beyond its brief. Yet many of the applicants would need special care. Might it be possible that at least one home should be available for those needing additional care and attention? William Stoate was determined that it should be done.

Precisely what suggested Bath as a likely site no one knows. Founded by the Romans, falling into ruin after the legions left, a squalid small town from medieval days through Tudor and Stuart times, it became the most fashionable resort in Britain in the eighteenth century. With the warm-toned stone from Ralph Allen's quarries at Combe Down there was built one of the most elegant cities in the country, graced by splendid palladian terraces and crescents on Lansdowne. In the last century a pleasant green space was opened out not far from these gracious houses and loyally named Victoria Park. Bath was the site of some of John Wesley's earliest open-air preaching. It was here that he had a notable encounter with the arbiter of regency fashion, Beau Nash; and to Bath, a century later, there was transferred the school he began in Bristol for preachers' sons. Kingswood School is now a public school of considerable note.

From the Methodist viewpoint, therefore, Bath had much to commend it—and, so far, there was no home in the West of England. William Stoate and the Langs began looking for a possible house. They found one overlooking Victoria Park—a run-down nursing home, going reasonably cheap. The Langs believed it had possibilities.

'You couldn't get more than five residents in here', countered Stoate. 'Look at the way that drain runs at the back!' They went and examined it. 'It would make any extension impossible.'

The Langs would not be put off. 'Ask the builders', they said.

The builders came, looked, measured and made up their minds. It could be done—and they did it.

Now Stratton House has twenty-eight residents, eighteen of them over ninety, and almost all the others over eighty. They are all frail, and most of them suffer from rheumatism, arthritis or heart-trouble.

'We're all females in this house,' said matron, 'except the grandfather-clock—and he doesn't give any trouble!' It is a necessary limitation, for here, in contrast to other homes, some of the residents are in rooms holding three or four beds, though they are discreetly screened. Alterations, however, are planned to accommodate a small number of men.

Because they are frail they cannot often go out, apart from specially-arranged outings. But they do not sit and do nothing; and the world comes in to them. After breakfast in bed they may often be found poring over 'Scrabble dictionaries' in the morning, and trying out their discoveries against each other in the evening. There is a service on Sunday afternoons, and once a month the local Women's Fellowship has its meeting at Stratton House, bringing tea for themselves and the residents. Large-print books brought by the librarian from the town library are changed fortnightly and are a godsend. A small 'shop' in the house is a compensation for not being able to go into the town.

Four other homes—at Woking, Leicester, Hull and Bowdon—were eventually to be opened to those needing special care, and Ipswich will provide a sixth. Bath pioneered a useful, if inevitably limited, type of home. Several of those who eventually found their way to one of these homes have already been residents in one of the general homes until they needed a measure of skilled nursing.

William Stoate, who succeeded Walter Hall as secretary, was already a retired minister. The Methodist Conference, indeed, was always to resist the appointment of a minister in full-time work to this task. With great goodness of heart and abundant energy he was a Somerset man who came from a milling family at Watchet. Both his father and uncle were millers and, after going to Taunton School, William served in the family business, milling grain and selling flour as a wholesaler before he entered the Methodist ministry. It was an early experience that gave him common ground with his treasurer, Mrs Lang, though the Stoate mills were small grain indeed compared with the Rank empire. He had considerable experience, too, in property management. The first part of his ministry was spent in the Home Counties but he then broke down in health and had to retire for five years. Coming back to the active work in 1940 he served in Devonport, Brixham and Tiverton—a part of England close to his heart—and he found special joy in opening the first West-country home in Bath.

As much as Walter Hall, he cherished the ideal that those who entered the homes should lead a full life. Few things made him angry, but one always roused his temper. That was when someone talked about the 'inmates' of the homes.

'Those who live in our home are *not* inmates.' His stature seemed to grow as his indignation rose. 'They are *residents*!'

Like Hall, and Richard Connell who succeeded him, he visited the homes regularly and came to know both residents and staff quickly and intimately.

Throughout his tenure of office the committee's main problem was lack of money, and Stoate was convinced that this was because Methodism as a whole did not value the homes fully. The income in 1950 was £47,000 and this had been stimulated by yet a third 'challenge offer' from the Joseph Rank Benevolent Trust. If the Church would raise £30,000 in three years, the Trust would add another £10,000. A brochure issued at this time, with a picture of Fulwood Park on the front, is headed

HUNDREDS
of applicants are waiting
—and sympathy is not enough!

Why should Methodism take any responsibility for these people? Was not the state doing all that was necessary? Clearly it was not. 'These are *our* people. We are *their* people. Should not the family, of which they have been faithful members, stand by them as the shadows lengthen and life's evening falls? Sympathy is not enough!' There was an element of pathos, almost of despair, in the leaflet. How much more than sympathy was Methodism at large prepared to offer? Had it not been for the 'Rank challenge offers' the income would have been far below what was needed to maintain the homes and plan for necessary extensions. In 1951 came a fourth offer from the Trust—a further £1 for every £3 raised, up to a total of £60,000 raised. It was to be the last offer of its kind for almost twenty years, though the Trust contributed with generosity to special projects.

The truth is that, in general, the appeal and value of the homes had not caught the imagination of most local churches which were now struggling through the aftermath of war. But though large gifts or donations were rare it must be recognized that there was a steady flow of contributions. Had this not been so the 'challenge offers' could not have been claimed. These offers *did* stimulate giving and, as the homes spread, knowledge of their work increased. Many of the gifts were from individuals, and were given sacrificially. Margaret Harwood, of the *Methodist Recorder*, insisted that 'little gifts make big totals'. The Flower Fund was increasingly used to pay tribute to good lives well lived. Local homes claimed local interest but most gifts came direct to the MHA headquarters. Nevertheless, financial stringency was to limit the things William Stoate longed to do during his term of office as secretary.

The lack of funds, however, did nothing to inhibit the steady flow of applications for admission—and the desirability of a professional approach to publicity and advocacy was not to be fully accepted for almost another ten years.

It must have touched Mrs Lang's heart to receive a cheque for £100 when the affairs of the Silver Band at Reigate, where she lived, were wound up. It came with good wishes for the work of the homes, in 1951. In that same year two new homes were to be opened. One was again in Stoate's own West-country.

Exmouth was sacked by the Danes and not really rebuilt until the nineteenth century. But Littleham Cross, a couple of miles from the Exmouth coast, has been a living parish for centuries—and in 1815, the year of Waterloo, a village girl linked the middle ages with the almost-modern world by walking in a white robe from church gate to church door, where she was excommunicated. It was the last public penance in England.

From a farmhouse at Littleham Cross the view extended across the country, over the valley to the hills beyond, and down to the river Exe. That farmhouse, suitably extended, is Moreton, the Methodist Home for the Aged. Once the home of the Walton Turners, it came to the MHA as a generous gift, reflecting the warm-hearted involvement of the family in the community for many years. In Exmouth they owned a departmental store which now has branches in other West of England towns, but the Turners had wider interests than their business. Active in Boys' Brigade affairs, as well as in promoting lawn tennis, they also founded and supported a convalescent home, Resthaven. When Mr and Mrs Leonard Walton Turner decided to move from their family home, Moreton, to a house on the moors they could think of no better memorial to their son, Kenneth, who was killed in World War II, than to present their home to the MHA. A tablet in the home records their generosity, their family tradition and their attitude to life.

> 'In past years God blessed the House of "Moreton" with much radiance. May his blessing continue to brighten the years of those who live here.'

That prayer is being richly answered.

Of its own type, a homely welcoming house in a not over-built residential area, Moreton is excellent. The decoration is light, the large lounge and dining-room both look on to the spacious garden, and from the residents' rooms, varied in size, the view of the country and the glimpses of the river are those which the Walton Turners loved .

Moreton has another charming feature, too. This is a cottage for that essential staff member of all the homes, the gardener-handyman. What makes this one different is that it was the gift of a resident, Miss Lavinia Elizabeth Carter, sister of a great secretary of the Methodist Christian Citizenship Department, the Rev. Henry Carter. She gave it, as a tablet on the cottage records, 'as a memorial to her family and in gratitude for eight happy years of fellowship in the Exmouth home'. Even more happily, it was built and occupied while she was still a resident.

Is Exmouth somewhat away from 'the stream of life', as Walter Hall once described an essential feature of the homes? Not at all. 'Life' is a local activity and many of the residents share in it very fully. An artist has his room full of Devon views, his own paintings. A minister cherishes indoor plants, but still preaches and exercises useful pastoral care amongst the residents. Two people go to a music group at the nearby teacher training college, Rolle College. Another goes to a weekly chess club—and he is over ninety. There is an ornithologist in his late eighties who walks the eight miles to Budleigh Salterton every week, cherishing this pleasant landscape, noting his 'sightings', and then comes home on the bus. Such people are very much a part of the 'stream of life'.

At Meriden the inhabitants will show you a tree which stands at 'the exact centre of England'. By contrast Leamington Spa, a few miles away, despite its grey Pump Room and a few good Regency buildings, is comparatively undistinguished. So, indeed, is Homewood at first sight.

On the Kenilworth road there stood a private hotel, and the baize notice-board still hangs on the wall in the hall. With long, narrow passages and too many steps and stairs it would not now be chosen for an old people's home. Yet it is all too easy to criticize with hindsight. In the 1950s Mr F. Johnston Carey, one of Hall's original committee, felt the need of a home in the Midlands—and Leamington was at the heart of England. Few local authorities' homes, at this time, were purpose-built or offered much in the way of privacy, convenience or amenities. To Midland Methodists, therefore, a hotel with single rooms already in existence must have seemed well worth buying. Not least important, there were adequate toilets and a not over-large garden. It is not far from the town. Through the years small extensions have been made.

Despite its physical limitations Homewood points up the truth that it is people, rather than surroundings, which make a home. Many now-frail residents still maintain a sharp interest in life and others have a close contact with it. Would one expect, in such a setting, to find a lady going to jewellery classes each week? Or to discover two Quaker sisters, both there for fifteen years, who had worked with a coal-miners' education project and still kept up with contemporary thinking by belonging to two libraries? Or to hear shrewd comments on dress from a lady six months off her hundredth birthday? Few local authority homes, however well-appointed, would have a retired minister who still went out teaching in a day-school two or three days each week.

Yet the heart of the home throbs more deeply than this, as a recent letter from a resident says very plainly.

'Old age is the best part of one's life. I am amongst friends who share the same sense of values; where all gather, if we wish, in the lounge at eight o'clock in the evening to join in singing and prayer at the end of the day. This, to me, is the most precious part of the day—to feel that we are at peace with one another at the end of the day, and at peace with God.'

Homewood, at Leamington, continues to prove its worth. But with the exception of a small home, Woodbank Lodge, which was preparatory to the main home at Woking, it was the last to be opened for four years.

8

One small office

Woking/Colwyn Bay/Lytham St Annes

Mrs Florence Lowe was a member of the general committee of the National Children's Home and was in its meeting when Walter Hall was asked to speak about his new project then in its earliest stages. Mrs Hilda Lang was then, and remained for many years, the treasurer of one of the NCHO's main fund-raising projects, the League of Light. Hall's words to the committee had a startling result. The committee, dealing with work amongst children, was so caught by his new scheme for the aged that it made a grant of the first £1,000 donation received by the MHA. But, in the long term, that committee had more important results. It lit Mrs Lowe's own enthusiasm, too.

Still energetic enough for someone twenty years younger, Mrs Lowe was in her eighties, though few people could have realized it. She at once got into touch with Hall, assured him of her interest and promised her support. The work of the MHA would have been in complete accord with her husband's wishes—he had died in the 1930s—and she was anxious to use his considerable fortune as he would himself have desired. They had contributed a steady flow of gifts to the National Children's Home. The Missionary Society was eventually to receive from her a legacy of some £200,000 which would be used to promote or amplify retirement schemes for ministers in overseas churches. She knew, too, that George Lowe would have been deeply sympathetic to the new Homes for the Aged. She saw to it that her own interpretation of his wishes was given free rein.

A daughter of the manse, she claimed vague acquaintance with the MHA chairman, Sir George Martin, because she had lived in some of the houses where he himself had lived. She became a teacher—with ideas of her own. Indeed, individuality was to characterize her whole life. George Lowe was a carpenter and he, too, had his own way of looking at things. On the Liverpool docks he saw one of the early refrigeration-ships arrive with meat from South America. Cold storage for meat? Surely there was a future in it—even, perhaps, a fortune? He was prepared to risk his money on the pioneering idea and the eventual outcome was the London Central Meat Company, and very considerable wealth for the Lowes. In Sutton Coldfield their generosity was quiet but consistent, though Henley and later Woking became Mrs Lowe's home. She always said that she left Sutton Coldfield because she had no wish to be fussed with the inevitable restrictions on her time if she became mayor!

Shortly before her husband's death they were discussing the future. 'We have done a great deal for the young', he said; 'now we ought to do something for the elderly. Those retired missionary ladies you're so interested in . . . some of them have nowhere to retire to when they come home. We ought to do something for *them*.'

The result was 'Little Woodbank'—her own name for what was properly Woodbank Lodge. This was a small house in the grounds of the large house she bought in Woking—where, untypically, she reported discovering a squash court which she knew nothing about when she purchased the house. This became the home for the 'retired missionary ladies' they had talked about. In 1952 it became the property of the MHA and, in the large grounds, a completely new home was to be built. But that was not done for another six years.

Mrs Lowe's interest in the MHA was not confined to Woking. She joined in the search for suitable properties and showed a keen interest in those already in use. Disturbed by the facilities at Bath, where the staff did their best for the frail residents with very inadequate cooking arrangements, she set out to provide ideal kitchen equipment when the material available was still very limited after the war.

Right through her eighties she visited the Westminster office frequently, to discuss what was needed and to offer her help—and advice—and usually bringing a packet of sandwiches with her. The office staff could recall being uneasy that, at the age of ninety, she should refuse their help to find a taxi outside the

Central Hall, preferring to do so herself. They later discovered that she had gone to the hairdressers, then to Guildford, where she was living, for a meal and an evening performance at the repertory theatre before going home.

She was gracious, practical, generous and refreshing; she was always determined and sometimes startling. What she had been she remained to the end, and she lived to within a few months of her hundredth birthday. The committee and the residents of the homes owed her a very great deal.

In 1952, when Woodbank Lodge took in its first residents, the MHA published its annual report. It could then claim 165 residents in its ten homes. They came from 112 circuits in thirty-two Methodist districts, and hailed from thirty counties. Limited though the distribution of the homes was, the net they cast was very wide.

But, at that same time, the waiting list had more names on it than there were residents. William Stoate, open-hearted but unable to be open-handed, was harder pressed by work and anxiety than anyone realized. Already there were demands for expansion, even in the houses which existed. Not only was the small home at Woking inadequate; the same was true of Wallington, the first home, too. Had it not been for the interest of the local committees, and especially of the local treasurers who were already proving themselves a second line of administrators, the task would have been impossible and the whole venture would have collapsed. Certainly the London staff could not have coped with all the demands and all the emergencies on its own.

The 1952 report used a photograph to make this plain, and to counter criticism of head office extravagance! 'How many people keep the headquarters going?' asked the caption. 'Not twenty, nor even a dozen', it went on. Then, directing the reader to a photograph with a couple of desks and some filing cabinets as a background, it put the answer in italics. '*Four!*' With William Stoate standing taller than the rest, it showed one other man, Bertie Winter, and two women, Miss Vera Purnell and Miss Lena Picking. William Stoate and Bertie Winter were not to have much longer in the office. But Miss Picking was to be there twenty years later, at the farewell to the chairman and treasurer, —a personalized symbol of the vitality, the resource, the dedication of the unseen and largely unknown members of the Westminster office staff who did so much of the essential but unpublicised work.

After a break of four years without a home being opened, mainly through shortage of money rather than any lack of suggested houses or locations, the programme seemed to be 'off the ground' once more. Homes were opened at Colwyn Bay in 1956, and at Lytham St Annes and Shirley in 1958. At that time, too, the new home took the place of Woodbank Lodge and a second house was bought to allow for extension at Wallington.

Of the new homes two were in the north-east. Apart from the home for frail residents at Bowdon, they were to be the last homes opened in the north-west for almost twenty years.

There is apt to be some confusion about 'dates of opening'. At the back of this book is a list of homes with the year in which the 'official' opening took place. For clarification it should be pointed out that residents have always been living in the home for several months before the official opening takes place.

The first new home was at Colwyn Bay.

Geographically, Colwyn Bay is in North Wales. Sociologically, many people would rate it an extension of Lancashire, Yorkshire and the Midlands! Welsh may be spoken in the shops, especially in the smaller ones, but north-country and midland accents are heard in the streets, and not only in the tourist season. A great many of the residents are English people who have retired to this part of Wales because of its sunshine record and, more specifically, because so many other English friends were there already. The English come as visitors to the Guild guest-house, Plas-y-coed (though few know that the name means 'the place in the woods') at Colwyn Bay, while others send their children to the two Methodist public schools in the same town, Rydal and Penrhos. True, there are large numbers of people who have never worshipped in English, done all their schooling in Welsh, and have a harp with pride of place in their sitting-room rather than a piano. But the thought of entering a Methodist Home for the

Aged in Colwyn Bay did not seem to elderly people in England like going to a foreign country—which, properly and proudly, it is. They had been there before, some of them very often. They were going amongst friends.

The period between 'thinking about Colwyn Bay' and actually opening the home there illustrates the apparently slow and certainly lengthy process which attends the opening of a home anywhere. For some time there had been the feeling that it would be good to have a home in that area. The process of searching for a suitable house may take years rather than months, and it did at Colwyn Bay. A likely place was finally found which was on the market—a large property on Llanerch road which had originally been two houses but which had been joined into one by a firm of doctors and turned into a nursing home. In July 1954 it was agreed to purchase it for £6,500. Alterations to make it suitable for its new use were estimated at £15,000. Compared with present-day prices both the cost of the house and the alterations seem absurdly small. In September that year it was agreed to proceed with plans submitted by a local architect to provide some thirty-four bed-sitting-rooms.

One year and eight months after this decision the house was opened.

The amount of work done by the head office in London, and especially by the secretary and his immediate colleagues—the vetting of possible sites and especially of the most likely one; the appointment of architects and the meticulous checking of every aspect of the plans; the costing, and often the adjustments as a result of the process; the watchful eye on the site development and the inevitable delays in building, electrical installations, decoration and the delivery of equipment; the thoughtful examination of the claims of probable residents—all these and many other things have to be carried forward alongside the constant supervision of other homes all over the country. It is not surprising that the general secretary and the administrator, in the twenty years that followed Stoate's retirement, found themselves 'on the road' for roughly half of every year. Above all, finding the right staff is the greatest headache, and often, because of its slowness, the greatest heartache, that is attendant on the opening of a new home. Behind every opening lies this long, tedious, detailed and often frustrating programme. In many cases it now takes longer than it did in the 1950s.

The opening of Astoria fell on Wesley Day, 24th May 1956. The chairman was F. Johnston Carey, who had been active in the acquisition of Homewood, at Leamington, and the opener was Mrs Lang. Her references were literary. The MHA was like the old woman who lived in a shoe; in terms of needing money they were like Oliver Twist—always asking for more. But her point was effective. There were some 600 people on the waiting list—and, unlike the old woman, the MHA *did* know what to do—open more homes.

Now with some thirty residents, Astoria stands above the quiet road, with leaping rockeries and alpine plants beside the path. The house itself has a touch of Edwardian whimsy in its gables and dormer windows. Inside there is no geometric or careful precision. Twisting passages—but few steps—give a permanent impression of 'something else round the corner'. It has disadvantages outside—there is little garden for residents to sit in and no parking space—but, within, it is homely. Would the residents not prefer to be in one of the new, purpose-built homes? 'Not me', is the assured reply from one old lady. 'This is more like our own homes than these modern, new fangled places!' In a lovely situation between two hills, with splendid sunsets and more than the average share of sunshine, this home in North Wales is a comfortable place to be.

When they share the sacrament of holy communion the residents have an oak cross on the table. Made by a resident of over ninety, he had stamped his name on the underside of the base. 'When I was an apprentice I *had* to do it—and I'm still not ashamed to put it there.' It is an attitude characteristic of many residents in all the homes.

The cost of bringing happiness to old age was already taking its toll of William Stoate. He had worn himself out in doing good. By the end of 1954 he was taken seriously ill, and was unable to carry the burden of responsibility any longer. A loyal and able minister, Richard Connell, who had himself retired early, was brought in to assist him. The expression of thanks at the opening of Astoria by 'the general secretary, the Reverend Richard J. Connell, B.A., B.D.' marked the first public emergence of a man who was to mean a very great deal, in a vastly changing world, to the MHA.

In 1860 an artist bought land from the lord of the manor at Lytham St Annes, on the north Lancashire coast, to build himself a house. Richard Ansdell was one of four Liverpool animal painters who all achieved fame, but he was never in the Richard Stubbs class and his pictures are not likely to fetch high prices at Christie's, except as Victoriana. Dogs, dead game, mountain sheep and Spanish goats nevertheless brought him a good deal of Victorian fame, and some fortune. He called his new house Starr Hills, with a reference to the starr grass that grew on the sandhills. But, though he gave his name to the immediate area, achieved some local notability and insisted that the local railway halt should be called Ansdell Halt, he did not stay long. In 1864, four years after he built it, he sold the house and moved to Scotland—nearer to the sheep and the game. In time the house came into the possession of Major William Henry Hincksman. A plaque in the hall records that his mother was a missionary in the West Indies. His wife was daughter to Samuel Broadbent, a missionary in South Africa. His granddaughters were women well known in Methodism and one, Sister Dorothy Hincksman Farrar, was vice-president of the Methodist Conference in 1952, six years before Starr Hills was opened as a Methodist Home.

In World War I Starr Hills was a convalescent home for wounded soldiers. In World War II it was a hostel for the women's services. Between the wars it had been a private school. But it is the Hincksman aura which remains. There is a sentence on a plaque in the hall with these words.

> 'Here men and women found help, hospitality and friendship in the name of Jesus Christ.'

Those phrases are very true again today.

Victorian though animal-painter Ansdell's house is, it is neither oppressive, opulent nor antiquated, and it has some real advantages. It is near the shops and the shore. There are two splendid conservatories, filled with plants and flowers, and a compassable garden with good lawns. Twenty-six forest trees rise above the gardens. It seems inevitable that the residents should be happy, in the spirit of the words in the hall. Apart from their own interests—'normal for people of their age', comments the treasurer—there is the pleasure of close contact with a very understanding church and circuit. Here is a home where many residents have local friends who come to visit them; where youth comes to provide entertainment; where the Young Wives visit regularly; and where those who come in from 'outside' are as much at home as those who live there.

And these 'normal interests for people of their age'? Pottery-making, evening classes, flower-arrangement groups, playing the harmonica. How refreshing to find elderly people with such 'normal' interests—and there are many other activities besides.

For Reg Spray, the lay administrator at the head office who joined the MHA soon after Richard Connell's arrival there, and who lived at Woking, it was a particular happiness that the new home at Woking was opened soon after he came into the organization. Woodbank Lodge, or 'Little Woodbank', as Mrs Lowe affectionately called it, intended by her for retired missionaries, had only been a beginning. Now, in 1958, the new building was opened. It had some distinctive features.

Up to now, in line with Mrs Lowe's own special interests, there have only been women residents, but alterations will make it possible to accommodate men also. Built amongst the woods, it was more quiet—and indeed more isolated—than any of the other homes. But if the 'stream of life' is some distance away, it has some very positive features. The main advance at Woodbank is that it was purpose-built, the first home to be so. The result is that it has only two floors and is well-planned. One aspect of this planning is that the residents' rooms are on only one side of the corridor; on the other are toilets, bathrooms, rooms where tea can be made; wash-rooms for personal laundry. Woodbank is still some distance in planning from private toilets in residents' own rooms—that was to come later—but it went a great deal further in purposeful design than any of the previous homes.

At the entrance is a delightful multi-coloured mosaic plaque of wild flowers, designed by the architect of the home, Mr Graeme Highett, and made by Poole Pottery 'to cheer the heart of all who pass through the door, that every month, every day, be it winter or summer, there is a flower to be found not far away'.

Some of that 'cheer of heart' is certainly to be found behind these doors.

Nowhere was that more evident than in one resident, well in her nineties, who was always 'the life and soul of the home'. Resolutely she refused to grow old. Widow of a distinguished Indian missionary, her memories of the past were vivid—and her interest in contemporary affairs intense. Tiny in stature she went up the stairs two at a time, refusing the lift 'because it was meant for those who were unable to use their legs'. She played the piano with great panache, though she could not see the music and did not need it. Nearly blind, within a few months of her hundredth birthday she still worked out chess-problems by touch; it was only a little while since she had given up reading Agatha Christie with the aid of a torch and two magnifying glasses. Almost completely deaf, she listened to what she could gather of the news each day on the radio. A 'character' in the fullest sense of that word, she always gave more than she took from others. With a joyous sense of humour and a deep fount of love, she was the epitome of all that is best in those who become residents in these homes and, at the same time, the justification for their existence.

It was at Woking that the first 'shop' was opened, to compensate for the distance from the town. Woking's example has been copied in several other homes, especially in places where the residents are frail and cannot easily go out to shop for their own needs.

9

The Wilderness transformed

Shirley

In May 1954, after William Stoate had fallen seriously ill as the result of his intensive labours and the anxious stresses he had known during his term of office as general secretary, the committee decided to appoint Richard Connell as his assistant. He was to attend at the Westminster office on three days a week, with a remuneration of 25s a day plus travelling expenses and, at his own request, his name would not be printed in any literature or included in the list of officers. By the following January he was invited to become general secretary, since it was clear that Stoate would not be able to continue his work.

Born in Luton, of a stalwart Primitive Methodist family, Richard Connell was accepted for the Primitive Methodist ministry and trained at Hartley Victoria College in Manchester. His academic ability led to his studying for a further year at a German university before serving in circuits at Bournemouth, Cambridge, Northampton, Loughborough, Leicester and Kettering. There were few of these places where he did not make and maintain friendships which were later to prove of value in his work with the MHA. His wife Phyllis came from Leighton Buzzard and, both on his own side and through her family interests, he gained a considerable knowledge of business affairs. This gave him an ability to talk to builders, contractors and quantity surveyors in terms which showed him to be no genial, other-worldly figure of the mythical parsonic type. Genial he certainly was, but he was entirely practical; never short of idealism, he nevertheless understood the hard realities of life amongst the developers as well as amongst the aged.

A serious car crash in 1933, after he had only been in his first circuit for a year, resulted in Mrs Connell suffering severe injuries, with an appalling number of broken bones, just as she was getting over pneumonia. Though she recovered, her health was precarious. During the war he was an officiating chaplain to the armed forces, as well as a circuit minister, but it was during that period, especially in Loughborough, that he came closely in contact with the problems of the elderly. Mrs Connell's health began to deteriorate after the war was over and the doctor gave Connell himself the option of changing his occupation or finding a place where his wife would be able to live quietly—if she were to live at all. He became a supernumerary minister in 1954 and moved to the south coast.

At the Westminster office of the MHA it seemed a providential retirement. Connell hoped to return to the full work of the ministry within a couple of years, with his wife fully recovered. The MHA could meanwhile use his considerable skills to ease the burden on William Stoate. It might make it possible for Stoate to return to work, better in health, and it would prevent Connell from having a gnawing feeling of frustration and his wife suffering any sense of guilt that he had had to retire after only twenty years of active ministry.

As things turned out, he was to serve as general secretary for twenty years and, for much of the time, his wife was sufficiently well not only to accompany him on many of his nation-wide itinerations amongst the homes but to be an effective partner in suggesting practical improvements.

Those years in the second half of the 1950s were full of 'firsts'—premium bonds were issued for the first time; the Queen made her first television broadcast; the first women life peers were created; Sir Vivian Fuchs completed the first crossing of Antarctica; three animals were the first living creatures to fly in space; the Russians took the first pictures of the back of the moon.

It was also the period when the first Methodist Homes were designed and built for their own proper purpose—at Woking and Shirley—instead of adapting existing houses.

But, for the new general secretary, there were a great many assessments to be made before any further advances could be undertaken.

How far could the MHA do anything in the least significant to meet the growing demands of the elderly? The most recent census before Connell took office showed that there were at least 750,000 widows and spinsters living alone in Britain. The projection was, that within twenty-five years, that number would increase to a million. It needed faith to believe that a few homes run by Methodism, largely for Methodist people, would do anything to solve the problem. In fact, though the intention had never been to solve any real measure of the problem but only to contribute to its solution, the work of the MHA was already influencing other groups and associations concerned with making provision for the elderly.

But to what extent could the home even meet the needs of the elderly within Methodism itself? There were only 216 residents when Connell came into the organization, and they would have to build quickly even to double that number. In fact, building was so effective that five times that number would be housed in Methodist Homes within twenty years. But it was plain that life in the homes was having an effect few people had predicted. Not only were the residents happy and relaxed but, because of this and also because of warmth and carefully balanced diet, they were living longer. It was not so many years previously that the old might be expected to live to seventy or seventy-five. Now, in the homes, the average was over eighty. In the home for the frail at Bath it was eighty-seven. And there were many over ninety.

The number of vacancies each year was considerably less than might have been anticipated.

How many new homes could be built—and how quickly? This depended entirely on the amount of money available . . . on how far Methodism was prepared to support the MHA with its annual income . . . on legacy income and its increase . . . on whether sources outside Methodism could be tapped. It seemed unlikely that the graph of income would rise very sharply. Yet the truth was simple—income rose as interest and knowledge spread. In 1950 the income was £47,000 and this was to rise, by 1960, to £98,000. It would have to do more than double in the following decade if it were to keep in line with the escalating cost of building and maintenance.

In the end, it did so—and more. By 1970 it was six times the 1950 figure.

What was of special interest was the legacy income. By the end of the 1950s it was gaining the benefit of those who had been sufficiently impressed to put the MHA into their wills. In 1950, when few people had heard of the MHA early enough to make it a beneficiary in their wills, the legacy income was £5,000. But by 1960 it had risen to £64,000. Within another fifteen years the growth was to be astronomical compared with those earlier years.

It would have been improvident to predict the continuing support of the Joseph Rank Benevolent Trust, despite Mrs Lang's interest. In fact, there was not to be another 'challenge offer' until almost the 1970s but there was a most encouraging gift of £5,000 to match an equally generous anonymous gift of £5,000 in 1956. That must have brought cheer to the new secretary—but still more encouraging was the steady stream of comparatively small but equally generous gifts which showed personal concern and sometimes sacrifice and at the same time evidenced the growing awareness of the MHA throughout Methodism.

There had been a vaguely hopeful idea of 'A Methodist Home for the Aged in every Methodist District'. That dream has not, even yet, been completely fulfilled, but, at that time, it was the gaps which stood out most poignantly. If building became possible, where should they move in? There were no homes in East Anglia; the South-East Midlands; the east coast; the North-East; the south coast (the most popular area for the elderly in Britain) apart from Bognor; none in Cornwall, South Wales, Scotland, or even London itself.

Alongside all these matters which needed careful thought was another pressure-point. The work in the office had broken Stoate; it must not be permitted to do the same to another secretary. More help was needed in the office itself.

'The man for the moment' and, indeed, for almost twenty years, who was prepared to change jobs and come to a task quite different from his own, was H. Reginald Spray.

Reg Spray was born in St Leonards-on-Sea and, like Richard Connell, he came from a Primitive Methodist background. His father, a grandfather and a great-grandfather had all been local (lay) preachers, and his father had been very active in his local church. Because both his parents died early he came to Woking to live with an uncle and aunt. At Woking Grammar School the headmaster was a Methodist who had served on committees with Walter Hall. But it was because his uncle, Mr Arnold, had a coal, forage and agricultural business that Reg Spray spent most of his early working life in that business. When he later left the business he moved to a company specializing in copper roofing—they were to provide roofing for the homes at Leicester and the Isle of Wight—and a knowledge of building came with his growing understanding of roofing techniques. It was from here that he came into the MHA, a little after the advent of Richard Connell, to share increasingly in administrative tasks.

Apart from the purchase of an additional house at Wallington to provide extension at Ryelands the only other MHA building to be added to the MHA list in the 1950s was at Shirley.

The Duke odf Devonshire held the patronage of the Anglican church at Shirley, not far from Croydon. Towards the end of the last century Croydon was no more than a market town with a famous school founded by Archbishop Whitgift, and Shirley was then a small village. The Duke installed as vicar a man for whom he had great respect, not out of regard for his spiritual qualities—though they may have been considerable—but because he was a gardener of eminence. Mr Wilkes, the new vicar, achieved fame far outside the parish. He became one of the most powerful secretaries of the Royal Horticultural Society, initiating its annual shows which developed into the Chelsea Flower Show. He was a founder of the famous Wisley Gardens, in Surrey. More than this, he developed a new strain of poppy, and named it the 'Shirley poppy'. Towards the time of his retirement he bought a piece of ground more or less opposite the church, full of trees, bushes and rank grass, built a house there and called it, appropriately 'The Wilderness'. Here he created a magnificent garden.

It was in 1934 that George Lewin saw a 'Sale' notice on the property. He bought it, transformed the garden yet again, and made it glow in early summer with azaleas and rhodedendrons

Lewin was in the building and development business, and was a leading citizen of the rapidly-expanding town of Croydon. Indeed, he became its major and his portrait in the red robes of office now hangs in the hall of what was once 'The Wilderness'. Then, in the 1950s, he and his wife decided to move, though not far away. They built a charming, appropriately-designed bungalow in the garden next to their home—and wondered what to do with the house they lived in.

The Lewins were great friends of the Halls, who lived not far away at Selsdon. They knew and valued his work and had kept in touch with it after Hall's retirement. Mrs Lewin knew precisely what they should do with their house.

'We ought to give it to the Methodist Homes for the Aged.'

At the age of ninety-five George Lewin is still involved in business. But his old home is full of happy, relaxed, retired people.

'But,' he commented, when he handed it over, 'it would never do to send old people into the wilderness! You'd better give it a new name. Call it after Walter Hall . . . he deserves it.'

So The Wilderness became Hall Grange—and a dignified portrait of this serene minister hangs in the lounge of the extended house that was once the Lewin's home. Hall's picture—the gift of his sons—was painted by Terence Cuneo, and Lewin's portrait in mayoral regalia by a Methodist minister, Herbert Waldron.

With its splendid extension making it possible to accommodate some thirty residents Hall Grange was opened by Lady Martin, the wife of the chairman, and the portrait of Walter Hall was received by Mrs Lang on behalf of the home.

Walter Hall himself was far from 'finished', as far as the work of the MHA was concerned. He seldom missed an officers' meeting at Westminster and still shared in interviewing prospective matrons and inspecting possible sites for future homes.

The intention was that Hall Grange should have a special care for the sick, and part of the premises were specially designed for their nursing and comfort. But, though it served its purpose, the difficulties of recruiting nursing staff has made it necessary to discontinue this part of the work almost entirely.

Few homes are lovelier in concept and reality than Hall

Grange. With only one storey above the ground floor it has a long, curving frontage extended from vicar Wilkes's original home. Inside, it is light-painted and bright. There are ironing and washing-rooms for the residents, and places were they can make tea and chat with their friends. It has an attractive dining-room and a splendid lounge with immense windows. But its chief pleasure is that not only the lounge but the window of every resident's room faces south across the great glory of the place—its eight acres of garden. True, George Lewin only gave four to the home and kept four for himself—but it would be hard to say which belongs to which. The only demarcation is not a fence nor a hedge but a vaguely discernible line—formed of azalea shrubs leading past the great rhododendron with a convenient seat standing near it.

Here is beauty indeed, and it is not surprising that residents spend long hours, especially in the spring and summer, looking away from their books and their embroidery, at the glory spread before them.

In the same year that Shirley was opened the first large extension was made to one of the early homes. This, appropriately, was at Wallington.

In 1955 the house next to Ryelands was bought for £6,500. Plans were drawn up to link the new house, The Moorings, with Ryelands by an extension which would include a new lounge and rooms for sixteen more residents, bringing its capacity into line with newer homes. The difference between buying old property and building new was immediately clear. The extensions cost £29,000. By today's standards the expenditure may seem trivial, but when the annual income was not much more than twice that sum the cost seemed frightening.

Today there are about thirty residents in a home which, for its first ten or more years, took only a dozen. The cost of maintaining the homes has, like building, risen unbelievably steeply. Residents have to pay a great deal more than they did when the Moorings was bought. But one elderly resident made her own comment on present-day economics.

'They say the treasurer takes most of your pension and there's very little left afterwards. But if you were a pensioner in your own home you wouldn't have *that* much left! Here you switch on your light when you want to. You have your meals, and your morning and evening drinks as well. There is warmth from your radiator. And you only have to go through your own door for company. Where would you get all *that* outside, and still have some of your pension left?

There are other advantages at Ryelands, though the old lady's personal comments apply to all the homes. Here church, shops, station, buses and library are only a few hundred yards from the door of the house. When Mrs Lang and her friends set their minds on Ryelands they chose better than they could have anticipated.

Now, another extension has been made and yet a further one is planned, this time with a second storey.

It was a minister's wife at Ryelands who read an article by someone who said that life was finished at eighty. She was incensed—for she herself was eighty-seven! She had always loved writing and, after she had poured out her indignation on her husband, she sat down to write.

'We thank Thee, O Father, for numberless things,
So much of happiness that every day brings;
For the blackbird that sings in our tree at dawn,
For the sunshine that brings out the chairs on the lawn . . .
For music, and friends, and children's faces,
And beauty that springs from unexpected places;
For contentment, a miracle that happens
Oft-times when the speed of life slackens;
Not grasping for unattainable things
But finding delight in simple things . . .
These gifts and a hundred others, no less,
Bring to old age deep thankfulness.'

The 1960s

Large extensions in progress

'Methodists are to be congratulated on being one of the pioneer bodies. . . . The approach of the Methodists and their concern for the older person as an individual, rather than concern with administrative convenience, is a shining example.'
—*Marjorie Bucke, Secretary of the National Old People's Welfare Council*

10

Building with a will

Dovercourt/Bury St Edmunds/Leicester

'Building with a will' was a significant, and doubly accurate, phrase as MHA moved into and through the 1960s. With its total income touching £100,000 and the legacy income reaching £64,000 the committee could offer thanks for a dramatically different picture from even five years earlier. It could begin, once more, to think of real expansion. The officers appointed by the Methodist Conference had shrewdly guided the committee through the first phase of tentative planning and a second period in which advance had been spasmodic and stress had taken its toll. Now both Sir George Martin and Mrs Lang were in a position to lead the organization forward with more positive assurance of backing from the church as a whole. The general secretary and the administrator were well able to mount the crest of the wave.

Neither Sir George nor Mrs Lang approached their task casually or with unrealistic optimism. Both were used to dealing with money, and equally assured in seeing that it was put to good use. They kept a penetrating watch on expenses in the office and on the way money was spent in buying, building, equipping and maintaining the homes. Extravagance was alien to them because they were aware of the cost that lay behind the thousands of gifts which made up each year's total income.

But their own care for the homes was matched by that of the head office staff. It was very small—most people would have said inadequate—to deal with the measure of business which occupied them at Westminster. Some of the early stalwarts were there no longer. Reg Spray's appointment, for instance, was due to the retirement of a man who had given astonishing service at the end of his working life—Bertie Winter. 'An incredible little man with an incredible memory'—so they remembered him. With little equipment provided to him and a bewildering mass of papers and files that seemed like chaos to a casual visitor he could, if the visitor or one of his colleagues demanded it, find the information they sought, either from his papers or from his phenomenal memory, in minutes and sometimes in seconds. If the office now had a better filing system, the foundation had been laid by him. But one contribution he made was of continuing importance. It was B. W. Winter who made the first approaches to local authorities for the supplementing of residents' payments in cases where their resources did not enable them to meet the payments due. This has been of tremendous help in the years that followed.

Miss Lena Picking would be in the office for another fifteen years. In the early days she kept the books, recorded the minutes, dealt with correspondence and provided the secretaries with information that was exact and relevant. As applications increased she was appointed to a position demanding tact, understanding and efficiency—'Applications and Vacancies'—and she filled it with skill and compassion.

In 1958 Mrs Dorothy Larbi came for three months—and is still there. She has been, officially, a receptionist, but over the years she has brought warmth to her welcomes, set nervous applicants at their ease, and sent overseas visitors away with a glowing appreciation of British hospitality. And all of them were welcomed, or sped on their way, with tea or coffee and a happy word.

It was in the middle of the 1960s that Herbert Bailey joined the staff. In the earlier period finance had been managed with the help of Messrs Hartley, Wilkins and Flew, accountants with strong Methodist connections who had their offices at the Central Hall, but the need for MHA to have its own finance department was increasingly evident. Herbert Bailey, from 1964, established the accounts department and took charge of it. He brought a caring love to the work which was typical of a local preacher deeply rooted in the life of his local church. By the time he suffered a severe illness and was off work for a period, a qualified accountant had become essential to a charity of this kind and Colin Smith, F.C.A. was appointed. When Herbert Bailey was able to return to the office he became the almoner, with responsibility for residents' payments—a task which involved him in a good many explanations whenever payments had to be increased and, at the same time, won him many friends amongst people whom he had never seen.

Already, by the beginning of this period, Richard Connell was 'Father' to those in headquarters and an increasingly familiar figure in the homes. He was travelling a great deal and, as the number of homes increased, was to spend something like half the year out of London. Both administrative and pastoral needs were considerable in the homes themselves and involved Spray in much the same amount of travel as they did Connell. The MHA has never been an organization in which 'London' is a long way off.

On this small staff, still to be housed for some time in the smallish rooms at the back of the Central Hall at Westminster and without any 'front entrance', there fell an increasingly heavy load of work. At last, the homes were beginning to expand rapidly.

Between 1960 and 1970 twelve new homes were to be opened, flatlets for retired staff established, and many of the older homes extended. In that period the staff expanded to a dozen, in addition to the officers.

The first new home of the decade was at Dovercourt, in Essex.

Old Harwich was a tightly-packed medieval town, with one of the earliest lighthouses in Britain. Even when it began to grow into a busy port nobody would have thought of it as a desirable residential town. Then, in the 1850s, the local MP decided to promote Dovercourt, a suburb of Harwich, as a coastal resort. On its parade, at the turn of the century, was a hotel at which King Edward VII was a frequent visitor. Here he entertained Kaiser William of Germany and many other guests besides, official and unofficial, and it had become the headquarters of the Royal Harwich Yacht Squadron.

One morning in the mid-1950s there was a phone call at the head office. A friend reported that the Alexandra Hotel was for sale. It was finally bought from Charringtons, the brewers, in 1959 and opened as an MHA Home in 1962.

The opening had a memorable moment. The first resident, a retired deaconess came—symbolically—to the foot of the steps and stood there with her suitcase. She was a short woman, and looked up at the distinguished ministers and laymen above her.

'You gentlemen don't surely expect me to carry my own suitcase up the steps, do you?'

The question was not in the script! Perhaps they did expect it, but there was no option. The suitcase was picked up and Sister escorted inside. The first resident was officially 'in'—and at ninety-three she is still there, and still preaching.

Dovercourt was a 'better buy' than either of the other hotels-turned-homes. In situation it was pleasanter that Leamington, for it faces the sea, while the residents are protected from the rigours of the east wind by double glazing, and there is constant interest in the traffic in Harwich Harbour and Parkstone Quay. In amenities it has more to offer than the earlier hotel-home at Tankerton for there is ample space inside and outside. Within, its spacious ground floor is fitting to 'the best, and most royal, hotel'. Outside, there are croquet and clock-golf lawns, a rose garden and wide flower borders. The transformation of the grounds was not easy. The hotel bowling-green had been removed during the war and, with concrete and hardcore, turned into a site for a barrage-balloon. This had been superseded by the hotel car-park. The Alexandra Hall attached to the hotel had been the only public hall in Dovercourt and there was at first some resentment at its removal, despite the fact that it was unsafe. But, after the residents arrived, the work went forward steadily, and the rose garden was a special interest to some of the workmen.

'This is a wonderful place,' said one of them to his mate, 'they feed you well, look after you when you're ill, and bury you in the garden when you die. Look—there's two of them.' He pointed to the names by two of the rose-bushes. 'A man and woman—Hugh Wickson and Mrs McCready!'

Many of the homes contribute to local life in various ways, but few have made more of a mark than Dovercourt. One resident makes clocks—grandfather clocks varying from 6 inches to 7 feet, clocks that work, clocks for ornament, clocks for jewel-cases, clocks for storage purposes. 'I've sometimes wakened up at four o'clock in the morning with all the measurements in my head, and just got up and jotted them down.' It is not surprising that he has won many commendations in local exhibitions, including the coveted 'award of merit'. But he is only one of many. For three years the residents, with the matron's encouragement, entered the Essex County Council Old People's Handicraft Exhibition, won the cup each year, and then won it outright. When a new cup was presented they won this, too—and went on winning it.

Elderly people do not go into the MHA homes to sit and wait patiently for a quiet end. They enter them to go on living—and some to begin living when they thought the time had come to give up.

One of the most interesting overseas visitors to Dovercourt was a Portuguese woman social worker from Lisbon. Anxious to stimulate the care of the aged in the Latin countries of Europe—she worked with the Gulbenkian Foundation for twelve years—she came to see what was happening in Britain. At the top of her list were the MHA homes—because she had been recommended to study them by a minister working in Angola! 'I wish I could do what they do,' she said of the staff, 'but to do work of this kind you need a much deeper faith than I possess.' It was a tribute worth preserving, and would apply to all the homes.

It may well be asked why there was such a resurgence of building in the 1960s, after the struggles of the previous decade. Behind this lay a widening of interest throughout Methodism and beyond it. Between 1960 and 1970 there was an increase in general giving of almost £200,000, so that it reached £282,000 in 1970. In the same period the legacy income was stepped up by £120,000, and rose to £180,000 in that same year.

'Building with a will' came to have a very real significance. It was a phrase that was used in MHA publicity which had suddenly taken on a completely new look. Until almost 1960 publicity had been thoughtful, caring and—without disparagement—amateurish and rather dull. What was needed was an approach that was appealing, novel, widespread and, above all, professional. This came with the appointment of Mr. H. Norman Spencer, of Vernon & Company of Liverpool, who was already entrusted with the public relations material of some of the other Methodist departments, including the Missionary Society.

Advertisements in the *Methodist Recorder* began to catch fresh attention. The MHA started to appear in the columns of the secular press. Then, in 1958, Norman Spencer introduced one of his favourite publicity devices—MHA was to have its own symbol. It was to be used and become familiar on every piece of publicity produced by the organization. There was sometimes criticism about so much new material, and sometimes of its high quality, but it quickly became apparent that 'spending money on advertising' was a sure way of 'bringing in more money', and often from unlikely sources. This was certainly reflected in the legacy income.

It may have seemed costly but it was attractive because it was interesting—and one publication, the 'MHA map', became very well known indeed. Showing not only the location of homes all over Britain on a good clear map, it also picked out with gay, coloured drawings many of the places of interest in the areas where the homes were set. In revised format, it is still in use.

In 1962, the year the map was published, there were 440 residents—but the waiting list was some 600. The demand for more homes was growing steadily.

In that year, with Sir George Martin in the chair, Lord Mackintosh, a Methodist peer, opened the new home at Bury St Edmunds. Appropriately, after nearly twenty years of indefatigable and imaginative leadership, it was named 'The Martins' after the chairman and his wife. It was the first home in East Anglia.

The motto of this charming town is 'Shrine of a King, Cradle of the Law'. There are lovely places in the city—the Theatre Royal is one of the three oldest theatres in England; the Guildhall is a gracious building; the Angel Hotel was featured by Dickens in *Pickwick Papers*. The cathedral of St James, now renewed and extended, is full of white light and ethereal spaces. But history begins much earlier at Bury. In 904 the body of the Saxon king, Edmund, was brought here for burial after his murder by the Danes, and his shrine was visited by hosts of pilgrims in the centuries that followed. The Abbey, 'Shrine of a

King', with St Edmunds tomb, became one of the wealthiest in England.

But why 'Cradle of the Law'? Because here, on St Edmund's Day in 1214, under the pretext of a pilgrimage, twenty-five barons gathered to swear allegiance to each other and plot the ensnarement of the king. By the high altar, now no more than ruined stones in the abbey garden, they gave final form to a new charter of liberty—the Magna Carta. Runnymede where King John reluctantly signed the 'great charter' the following year, is shown to tourists as the place where British liberty was born—but Bury is the place where it was conceived.

When Henry VIII dissolved the monasteries, threw out the monks and stole their sumptuous treasures, the abbey of Bury St Edmunds began to fall into decay. Its stones were taken to build farmhouses while the abbey's vineyards, across the rippling little river Lark, were overrun by weeds and bushes. It was in these vinefields, then no more than rough ground, that Richard Connell, bringing his son to the Methodist school, Culford, saw an attractive site for an East Anglian home. The local minister began a careful, private investigation and initiated equally unpublicised negotiations. Lady Phyllis Macrae, the landowner, was prepared to sell it but the city fathers were unhappy to see any development on such a site. It might conceivably spoil the view for visitors to the abbey. In the end there was agreement. The home was built low, so that it slips into the site of the vinefields—but not so low that the residents do not have a splendid view of the abbey grounds. A bridge was provided so that they had access to the grounds and could take a short-cut to the town streets just beyond them. A plaque bears tribute to Mrs Godfrey of Luton, wife of an alderman, 'whose last wish was for a Methodist Home for senior citizens in East Anglia', and signifies their generosity.

There is little reason for MHA residents to be bored. Here at 'The Martins' the local committee arranges outings in the summer and these include an annual visit to Alexandra House at Dovercourt, while the Dovercourt residents make a return visit to Bury. There are regular entertainments—never too long—each fortnight throughout the winter, with music, films, choirs, slides and other activities. In addition there is an annual 'Invitation Day' when one circuit in the District is specially invited to visit the home. The chairman of the District presides. There is a prominent man as speaker, whose wife opens the sale of goods made by the residents or provided by local ladies and churches. The residents themselves form a choir. Each year, for a growing number of people, 'The Martins' is put on the map.

This was a period when the elderly were beginning to be taken more seriously by the local authorities, as well as by voluntary groups and associations. In 1948 local authorities had owned and managed only sixty-three 'small homes', and the transition from the old workhouse was then still going slowly. By 1960 another 1,121 had come into existence—though it must be noted that such a figure, apparently encouraging, meant less than 100 homes a year opened throughout the whole country. Many of the older homes owned by local councils or private charities were still pre-1900 buildings and, though they had large gardens and imposing drives, offered little in the way of amenities or privacy. It was still too common for old people to be huddled together in large common-rooms, and forbidden to go to their own smaller rooms or dormitories during the day unless they were ill and confined to bed.

True, local councils' homes were being built with more imagination, though there were still too few concessions to privacy. Even in a typical but good forty-resident home only half the residents were in single rooms while eight were in four-bed and ten in double rooms.

It is undeniable that the MHA was still a pioneer in the care of the elderly, even at this period. In too many cases the valuable Old People's Welfare Associations were still struggling against popular prejudice and general inertia.

Once more the central committee of the MHA was being pressed to offer more accommodation to the frail. Out of fifteen homes there was only one in this category, at Bath. In 1963 a second home for such residents was opened, at Leicester. More accurately, it is in Oadby, some distance from the city itself.

Aigburth, a large private house with considerable extensions, is situated in a very quiet residential area full of spacious houses, tree-lined roads and large gardens. Its main disadvantage, a considerable distance from shops and public transport, is mainly felt by the staff—and in the recruitment of staff—rather than by the residents themselves who, in the main, are too frail to venture out very far on their own. The equipment is designed to ease the work of those who must care for people who cannot care for themselves—though not all are by any means so limited as this—and the lift is large enough to accommodate walking-frames and wheel-chairs.

The matron in such a home must have nursing skills and experience. All rooms have emergency bells—this has become standard in most homes—and two-way radio communication with the matron. The matron's office has a board for registering emergency calls—and, from time to time, there *are* emergencies. Occasionally someone falls. Someone gets stuck while dressing. A resident may become fearful and need comfort. 'Calm, competent and caring' are the qualifications for those who work amongst the frail.

Next door to Aigburth are halls of residence for the University of Leicester. The young are more of a tonic than medicine for the elderly. Students 'adopt' residents and visit them regularly. They take Saturday morning prayers. They offer practical help in the house by way of 'odd jobs'. And if, in one resident's words, 'they do have noisy parties next door sometimes, they make up for it by the real interest they take in us'.

The Aigburth residents may not like parties, but they live a full life of their own. 'I have yet to go into a room', comments the matron, 'and find its occupant idle.'

11

Thanks a million!

Hull/Isle of Wight/Scarborough

1963 was a historic year for the MHA, and this was symbolized by a widely-distributed leaflet. Across the front, with the MHA symbol and a gigantic 'pound' sign, were the words: 'Thanks a Million!'

By that year over £1 million had been subscribed to the Methodist Homes for the Aged.

'This', stated the leaflet, 'is an investment in human happiness.'

In that year the investment was to grow rapidly. One home, at Leicester, had already been opened and three more were to follow. Of these the one which undoubtedly gave great personal pleasure to Mrs Bartlett Lang and her family was Willersley House, at Willerby, near Hull.

Built at the end of the nineteenth century by a well-known East Yorkshire family, the Smithsons, the house had changed hands several times and, when its last owner decided to sell, local Methodists felt it might well suit the purposes of the MHA. At first there was little enthusiasm in London, where a good many sites were being investigated. Indeed, when it came on the market it was offered to the University of Hull, who declined it as being too far from the city for student accommodation. Not until the chairman of the District, the Rev. F. Pratt Green—the most prolific and perhaps the best of modern Methodist poets—visited it with its original 'discoverer' was the suggestion considered with any real seriousness. After that, things moved more swiftly. The property was bought, repaired, extended and made ready for residents needing more than ordinary care.

Opened with most of the necessary adaptions already completed, it is a warm, welcoming and dignified house in which comfort is the keynote. The eighty-year-old magnolia tree in the garden was planted when the house was built, but most of the other attractions are more recent. There is a lily-pond in a sunken garden at the front of the house, and another sunken pond and garden have been created in the centre of the newly-built wing, on which residents can look down from their wide-windowed corridor upstairs.

Not far away Joseph Rank was born, and in Hull he established the milling business which was to make his fortune and, at the same time, make possible his great generosity. It was fitting that the new home at Hull should be linked with his memory. Willersley House was the name of the house where he had lived and where Mrs Lang, with her brothers and sisters, had spent their early years. It was happy and right, therefore, that Mrs Lang should open this new Willersley House. Indeed, the home was largely the creation of the Rank family—a gift of £50,000 from the Trust had made it possible.

In the 'quiet room' is another link with the family. On the wall hangs a large embroidered Maltese cross which was made by Mrs Lang in the 1930s. An inscription states that it used to hang in the dining-room of their Reigate home and was 'miraculously saved from German bombs in 1940'.

Here, as at Leicester, considerably more demands are made on the staff than in most homes. Because the frail need extra care three workers share night duty during the week. At Willerby, however, which used to be a small village but is now more closely linked with Hull, shops and church are only five or ten minutes away. There is a good deal of visiting by church members and residents are invited into friendly homes. They are taken to church by car—this is something that happens in connection with all the homes—and the outside world is brought in, especially by young people. The local Guides come in on Friday evenings and, during an August holiday-club for children at the church, each of the three age-groups catered for visit and share in the life of Willersley House.

A glance at the list of residents shows a position that is fairly typical. Only three residents are in their seventies; four are over ninety; and twenty-two are in their eighties. But it is perhaps unusual in having one lady of 103—and at her birthday party the youngest of her relatives to be present was seventy-nine.

It is probably through reading the 'minutes' of committees that one gains the simplest over-all view of what is happening in any organization. This is true of the homes belonging to the MHA.

Most homes have a 'social committee'. Quite distinct from the 'Home Committee' which is the committee of management, the social committee consists mainly of women from the area who co-operate with the matron and usually with the treasurer in running coffee mornings, sales, entertainments and so on. Such a committee is optional, but its value to the matron may well be considerable.

The 'Home Committee', on the other hand, is established as part of the constitution of the MHA. Its principal officer is the 'treasurer'—and the minutes of any Home Committee show how inadequate is the title. He is, in fact, much more truly the local 'administrator' and is in constant touch with the head office at Westminster. The chairman may well be the local minister or the chairman of the District. The Home Committee meets twice a year and the secretary or the pastoral director will be present.

One set of minutes will serve as an example of what happens in any of the Home Committees and illustrate the breadth of their responsibility. In this case the chairman was the local minister.

The committee included six women and five men, as well as the secretary from London. The bulk of the business was presented by the treasurer. It consists, according to the minutes, of a detailed report of the activities of the home; a careful presentation of the accounts (which were closely examined and questioned); a survey of repairs, maintenance, decoration and equipment; a summary of devotional life in the home; a report by the matron (especially about residents' health); and a close look at staffing problems.

A few items from the minutes exemplify the way in which the Home Committee is concerned with all that occurs.

During the year five residents had died, and thus five vacancies had been created for new residents. None had occurred for other reasons.

Entertainments had included church, children's and male voice choirs; a carol concert by a local school; a bell-ringers team;

colour slides and films and—the highlight—a pantomime by the Young Wives Club.

Devotions, apart from evening prayers taken by residents themselves, had been led by ministers and lay preachers, young people and a police group. The church Women's Fellowship had met from time to time in the home, and tape recordings had been specially useful.

Official visitors, outside Methodism, came from the city Welfare Department and, less frequently, from those running other voluntary homes and looking for adaptable ideas.

Spin-driers and equipment for the residents' tea-bars, equipments for residents confined to bed, bathroom aids for those needing help with washing and a good many smaller items had been purchased by the matron out of the funds raised by the year's coffee mornings, which had been greatly helped by members of the committee and from local churches.

There were reports to be considered from the chief officer of the local fire brigade about fire precautions; and others about the rising cost of light, heat, food, repairs and decorations. Tributes were paid with great warmth to the staff, and especially to the matron and her residential colleagues, and to the gardener/handyman (a key figure in all the homes) not only for maintaining part of the garden in beauty and another part in the prolific production of vegetables, but for his work in decorating rooms, executing running repairs and a dozen other tasks.

To peruse such minutes with imagination is to be made aware of the immense amount of work which the running of any of the homes entails; of the stress under which the staff must live from time to time; of the invaluable voluntary service given by a comparatively small group of people, and in particular by the treasurer; of the professional competence and skill made available through the London headquarters whenever it is needed. But, above all, in such a set of minutes there is the reflection of responsible caring which is implicit in all the homes.

The third home to be opened in 1963 was on entirely new ground—in the Isle of Wight. John Wesley wrote, after one of his visits to the island: 'I never saw a more fruitful, or more pleasant, country.' Many annual visitors would say the same, and would add equally complimentary comments about the freshness of the air, the peace of its rolling landscape and the welcoming quality of its people. Apart from its seeming remoteness from the mainland—the ferry does not really take long to cross the Solent—the island had all the advantages for happy and relaxed retirement that the MHA sought. But was a house available, suitable in size and setting, sufficiently near to town or village, shops and church?

At Colwell, near Freshwater, was a charming house which had been in use as a small private hotel. Colwell Bay was only a short distance away, and the sea could be seen from some of the upstairs windows. Totland and the Needles were not far and the village of Freshwater, where Tennyson lived for thirty years, was easy of access. In time this house came into the possession of the MHA. Miss Wanstell, the sister of a previous owner, herself commandant of the Red Cross, was delighted that this should be so and was greatly interested in the home which was given the name of Green Meadows. Her picture stands on a table in the lounge, for she was a warm friend in the early days.

No home has a stronger sense of community than Green Meadows, and the visitor will easily sense the enjoyment that characterizes its life. The open-plan lounge-dining-room can easily be converted into an area large enough for concerts or entertainment—and is the right size and shape, too, for the programme which the residents put on for themselves on Boxing Day. The well-designed first floor has strategically-placed 'bays', near the tea-making bars, with easy chairs where residents can sit comfortably and chat with each other. The picture-windows in the bays offer views of the garden and the sea. This pattern of informal sitting-out bays—a new feature introduced about this time—as well as private bed-sitting-rooms and public lounges, adds an extra dimension to community life.

As in other homes, the residents like to share in adding to the comforts of the house. This accounts for 'Petticoat Lane'—a stall which exists throughout three months of the year to raise funds. But the 'funds' are not reserved exclusively for immediate and local needs. Amongst other thoughtful contributions to a wider needy world the residents have adopted a thalidomide boy. The world breaks in, too; not least through the local Guides and Brownies. The District Guide Commissioner makes herself responsible for 'different-every-year' Christmas decorations, with the help of Guides from Freshwater and Totland, and the Brownies give immense joy by bringing Mothering Day posies and birthday cards.

On the table in the lounge is another photograph, alongside Miss Wanstell's, of a gentle-faced woman with kindly mouth and thoughtful eyes. The face would be unknown to almost everyone in Methodist, but most Methodists—and many others as well—have known her pen-name for nearly sixty years. This is 'Margaret Harwood'.

It was she who opened Green Meadows in April 1963, and the chairman, appropriately, was Eric Pigott, the editor of the *Methodist Recorder*. She lives not many miles away.

During World War I Sybil Haddock—for that is her real name—contributed some stories to the *Primitive Methodist Leader*. As a result the editor, the Rev. George Bennett, offered her a weekly space which quickly took shape as a correspondence column. When he urged her to 'keep your identity secret because a bit of mystery helps' she settled on the name by which, in journalism, she has been known ever since. From those early days, through the amalgamated *Methodist Times and Leader*, which was begun in 1932, and then in the *Methodist Recorder* with which it was united in 1937, 'Margaret Harwood' has kept in touch with an incalculable number of readers, and not all of them have been women. Her column only ceased in 1975 and, from the beginning, she received a steady stream of letters.

'People' always claimed her fullest interest, as her column has shown . . . people in need, or in trouble; people with problems of belief or behaviour; lonely, awkward, hurt people; married or unmarried, older or younger. It was perhaps inevitable that, with a journalist's eye and her personal sense of compassion, Walter Hall's early attempts to do something for the elderly and lonely people of Methodism should make an immediate appeal to her. The general committee meeting in 1945, with the homes hardly established, mentioned the success of her first appeal on their behalf. From that time onwards the homes were a recurring theme in her column. The result was a flow, and sometimes a flood, of gifts through the post. She was the sort of person who could hardly wait to read her letters, and she went to the post office herself, with her own case, rather than wait for the postman. She was equally unconventional with the gifts she had received, so that Reg Spray, paying a call on Green Meadows, found himself with a large brown-paper parcel thrust into his hands on his first visit to Margaret Harwood. It was full of money—postal orders, cheques, stamps, money in every form—received by Margaret Harwood from her readers for the homes.

Her early appeals soon became crystallized in the annual Christmas appeal through the columns of the *Recorder* and from this source she has raised many thousands of pounds—tens of thousands, indeed—for the funds of the MHA. In many cases the response was spontaneous, a wish to share with others; but there were many people whose gifts were sent in gratitude for the counsel or encouragement this compassionate journalist has given them in difficulty, sorrow, bereavement or personal loss. She herself was to suffer the loss of her daughter in a car crash soon after they had planned and built the bungalow they were to share together.

But Margaret Harwood's contribution to the MHA was not solely in raising money. She did a good deal to encourage the right kind of woman, with the right qualities and qualifications, to offer for service in the homes. It was fitting that, a few years later, the new home at Cramlington, in Northumberland, at the extreme end of England from her own island home, should be named Harwood Court.

A year after its opening Green Meadows had an unusual visitor. In his yellow robe he was indeed conspicuous, for Bhikku Vinita was a Buddhist monk from Ceylon. Brought up in a Methodist family and educated at a Methodist college he had nevertheless found his own peace in Sri Lanka's traditional faith, and was in charge of the London Buddhist Centre. Interested in the care of the aged in his own country, where a few homes already existed, he sought permission to visit the Methodist homes to study their work. He would have been prepared 'to sleep in a shed, or some quiet place', but in fact he was a welcome and interesting visitor who brought a new awareness of the world with him.

Though Vinita was a far more exotic figure than most visitors there have been many overseas people who have sought out one or other of the homes, sometimes from interest kindled by reading of the work they are doing and the possibility, like Bhikkhu, of learning lessons for their own circumstances. In addition to the Americans, Australians, New Zealanders, Canadians and South Africans, who might have been expected, others have come from European countries, including Russia, from Africa and Asia and Central America. Not so long ago there were visitors from Japan who came officially to examine the work of the MHA in order to introduce pioneering programmes of the same kind in their own country.

The last of the homes opened in 1963 was the result of a telephone conversation which Sir George Martin had with his friend Sir Henry Price. Sir Henry was a millionaire Yorkshireman, a great benefactor of his county, who had established the Fifty Shilling Tailors many years before. As Sir George recalls the conversation it was as blunt as only Yorkshire friends could be.

'I like your Homes for the Aged, George, I think I'll give you one.'

Sir George was honest. 'You're opening your mouth a bit wide, Henry. It will cost you £50,000!'

'Don't be insulting! Do you think I haven't got £50,000 to spare, George?' After a pause he went on. 'Go on, lad. Get it built. And I want it in Yorkshire.'

The result was Priceholme, in Givendale Road off North Leas Avenue in Scarborough. But, though he gave the money and gave his name to it, Sir Henry never saw the home. He fell ill before the opening and did not recover.

Scarborough is a lovely seaside town and probably the favourite resort of Yorkshire people. Already familiar to many of those who came as residents, to some it was the very place they would have chosen to retire. Near to the sea, with shops reasonably close and a new Methodist church on the other side of the road, the situation of Priceholme has much to commend it. But the home has much more that is attractive. A new-built home, not an adaptation of an old house, it has two storeys and two residential wings. The warm yellow stone and rich brick give it a mellow tone outside, and the glass walls of the main entrance corridor disclose an enclosed patio with interesting plants and a sense of space. In the main lounge is an attractive fireplace built of the same stone as the exterior of the home. The furniture in the dining-room was the gift of Sir George Martin.

It is no surprise that the residents are both happy and active, and one group has repaid something of their own good fortune by providing help for people far away and much in need. These are some half-dozen or more workers who have knitted blankets for refugees in Algeria, Bangladesh, Jordan and other places. That the blankets reach the people who really need them they are sure, for they have had letters in reply.

It has been said that one of the most important staff members in any home is the gardener-handyman. It is he who responds to calls for practical help from the matron or the treasurer. In most cases he is either more handyman than gardener, or vice versa, but occasionally he excels at both. This is the case at Scarborough, where his practical facility in decorating or painting is matched by equally high skill in creating beauty in gardens. In the hall at Priceholme hang certificates which bear authoritative testimony to the creativity behind the gardens the residents so much appreciate. The 'Britain in Bloom' competition has a number of categories and one of them is for 'a private garden open to the public gaze'. For this, Priceholme won a plaque, and the prize certificates in the hall are dated 1971, 1972, 1973 and 1974. Even Falmouth, which has won awards in the same competition at Langholme, can hardly better this.

12

Going too fast?

Wolverhampton/Muswell Hill/Hitchin

By the end of 1966 nine new homes had been opened in six years —though the planning for the earlier ones had been begun in the 1950s. In addition, four more were scheduled by 1970. Was the organization over-stretching itself? At the time Scarborough was opened (and this had been made possible by Sir Henry Price's personal generosity) there was a sense of relief at the head office that some of the slack of the 1950s had been drawn in, and that more of those on the waiting list could look forward confidently to 'a home in a home'. Throughout the country, too, there was an awareness of achievement. The income rose because there were nationwide signs of 'things being done'. In terms of giving, new homes meant the encouragement of new money.

Within a few years, however, there was a new note of questioning about the rate of expansion. When Wolverhampton was opened in 1966 there had not been a new home since 1963, but Muswell Hill and Hitchin were opened in that same year.

However slowly things had gone ten years earlier, were they not now moving too fast?

By 1965 the accommodation in the homes had risen to 565. But the waiting-list now had 633 names!

It was about this period that the age of entry was raised to seventy. This was not only to control the waiting-list but also because fewer people wanted to enter the homes before that age. Yet even with the raising of the entry age the waiting-list gave acute anxiety to the officers. The homes opened in 1963 had added about 100 more rooms, but it seemed that as more people went into the new homes even more people applied for consideration.

Despite this, there *was* criticism that too many homes were now being opened. The tension came because those who were continually being pressed by very real need, as expressed in sometimes pathetic letters, felt it unreasonable to call a halt. The criticisms fell into two main groups.

There were some people who thought it wrong to spend money on new homes when, in older ones, money was needed to bring the accommodation for staff and residents, as well as kitchen equipment and amenities, up to date.

Others recognized the claims of applicants who had waited for years for a place, but believed the situation would not be eased by building new homes unless, at the same time, there was an assurance that they would be fully, or at least adequately, staffed.

No one recognized the validity of these arguments more than the general committee and the officers themselves. In reporting to the 1966 Conference the general secretary wrote: 'We are not alone in this problem of staff. We hear of voluntary homes having to close, not from financial failure but through shortage of staff.' The problems of similar organizations, nevertheless, offered cold comfort to the MHA, and the passage of time only seemed to exacerbate the disability from which all such associations suffered. In 1969 the general secretary was still in trouble. He had to report on a home which had been newly built: 'It is beautifully built; the equipment is there; but we dare not open to admit residents who are already waiting because there is no resident cook.'

That difficulty had to be met in many homes by engaging non-resident cooks, and this seemed a backward step. But a non-resident matron in a home for aged people would be a contradiction in terms.

One man who had his own ready reply to the attitude of 'no more staff, no more homes' was John A. Bates of Wolverhampton. He had begun a small family footwear business in Wolverhampton and, over the years, had expanded it and opened new branches in other towns.

'If I always waited until an old shop were fully staffed I would never open a new branch at all!'

From a successful businessman it seemed a realistic attitude. He was sure, too, that only the likelihood of new homes being opened caused donors to include the MHA in their wills. 'Stop providing new homes and you withdraw the incentive to give!' The dilemma was real, but the waiting-list was imperative. And, so far as Wolverhampton was concerned, money was not to be a major problem.

Mr Bates had been happily married for fifty-four years, and forty of them had been associated with the Newhampton Road church in Wolverhampton. When Mrs Bates died her husband wished to offer some gift to Methodism in her memory. But what should it be? He did not believe in 'endowments' to local churches—'it keeps them open when they should be closed'—and he responded immediately to the suggestion of the Rev. Brian O'Gorman, the chairman of the District, that nothing would be more appropriate than a new home for the aged in the town they loved. If a site could be found Mr Bates said he would gladly give £50,000. O'Gorman and Norman Bates, the son of the donor, spent an afternoon a week for three months trying to find a suitable place, and eventually came upon a house in Ash Hill. Richard Connell visited it on the way back from Conference in July. The price was £13,000. The treasurer, Mrs Lang, was very uneasy. No previous site had cost so much and it seemed a very high expenditure in the mid-1960s. Eventually however, with the agreement of Sir George Martin, the house was bought.

Mr Bates and his wife Blanche had gone to Lucerne on holiday in 1921 and, as a result, had called their new home Engelberg. That name was now transferred to the MHA home to preserve old associations as well as the memory of Mrs Bates.

Set in a cul-de-sac at Compton, a few miles from the city centre, Engelberg is a one-acre site with a bus-stop at the end of the road. Five miles from the Shropshire border the air is clear and clean. Its thirty residents enjoy the spacious front garden, with its cypress trees and conifers, but find plenty of opportunities of 'getting out'. Many go out frequently, and there is a car service, as usual, to take them to church if they wish. But. with Shropshire countryside so near, there are opportunities of going farther afield, especially in the summer, with outings arranged to Ludlow, Craven Arms, Church Stretton or Cannock Chase—and a willing church at the other end to provide tea and sometimes entertainment.

Yet these elderly people do not rely on others to provide them with interest. They find their own occupations, from going out to a bridge club or a club for the deaf to playing scrabble or making furniture.

The happiness and relaxed good fellowship of those who had already found a place in the twenty-four homes which were now open only underlined the dilemma of whether to open yet more, or to call a halt. But, in terms of practical politics, there were already new homes being planned and sites being examined. It would not be as easy to stop as critics might imagine. Personal generosity in relation to the provision of actual sites for building —a growingly expensive part of planning for the future—would not be stemmed. It was essential to step up the recruitment of residential staff, and linked with this was the extension or modernization of accommodation in the older homes. These things would receive increasing attention—but the provision of more homes would continue.

Not all who applied for entry were Methodists—though the majority certainly were. It was impossible to staff the homes with Methodists, too. To what extent was the word 'Methodist' in the official title of the homes restrictive? To some people it appeared to have a forbiddingly denominational ring about it.

Some restatement of facts is important. The homes were begun by a Methodist minister to relieve the last years of Methodist people, at a period when care for the aged was minimal and sometimes heartless. It was the Methodist Conference which had established them, and which, by law, controlled them. As well as offering a type of life acceptable to the majority of those who entered them, this undergirding authority of the Methodist Conference also guaranteed their maintenance and continuance, in great measure.

Applicants had to assure the head office that they would fit into a community where values were high and would refrain from things which would 'upset' other residents. Alcohol, for instance, would not be permitted on the premises, though not all residents would necessarily be total abstainers. There was a Methodist atmosphere and ethos which has been maintained from the beginning.

None of this, however, has determined a denominational attitude in terms of support, residents or staff. Much of the money, at least in legacies, has come from non-Methodists. A good deal has come from sympathetic non-churchgoers and even non-Christians. The Jewish community has often been open-handed. Sympathy with the aims of the homes has been more significant to the donors than any interest in Methodism itself.

The majority of residents are, in fact, Methodists or have had Methodist links through their families. But in most homes there will be found representatives of other branches of the Church. Anglicans, Quakers, Baptists, and others bring their own experience which is of value to the whole community.

This is even more true of the staff. There has never been a rigorous policy of 'Methodists only', and it would certainly not have worked if there had been. It obviously makes a considerable difference if the residential staff share, as well as sympathize with, the Christian faith of those they will have in their care. They will not be embarrassed in common acts of worship—and indeed will be more able to see the necessity for them—and will be able to respond to residents' personal approaches and conversation. This is particularly true for matrons and assistant matrons who have the most intimate association with them—but other residential helpers, often quite young, who have a clear Christian commitment have brought great joy to their elderly friends. In fact, even in the senior staff, there are wide variations of churchmanship, though Methodists predominate. When it comes to the point, however, denominational allegiance is never valued above the essential qualities of understanding, professional skills, compassion and the ability to work with residents and staff while avoiding any obvious 'management' of them.

It cannot be reiterated too often that the quality of a home depends on its staff and, above all, on its matron.

Nor can it be stated too frequently that staff recruitment is the most urgent problem faced by the MHA, and that in this work will be found a personal sense of fulfilment and satisfaction which is not easy to achieve in many professions or vocations.

The wide variety of religious background amongst the staff is matched by the greatly varied professional experience of, for instance, matrons and assistant matrons. Some come from nursing and some from the service of the church. There are widows who have, by and large, been housewives, and there are ex-missionaries. Some have worked in 'social care' of one kind or another—in the prison service, for instance, or in public welfare. One was a highly paid computer programmer who gave up a lucrative position to find vocational satisfaction in 'working with people'. Indeed, it is sometimes the case that experience of a very different occupation brings a valuable freshness of approach to the task they take up in the homes.

For more than one generation the name of Guy Chester was known throughout Methodism. His grandfather was a minister of the United Methodist Free Churches; his father a London layman who held most of the lay offices in the church. Harold Guylee Chester himself inherited their independence of judgement and their loyalty to the church but added his own creative ability and practical organizing skills. Early business success as an underwriter led him to high responsibility at Lloyds. But his activities were always coloured by an interest in international affairs. He was deeply committed to the League of Nations Union and, later, to the United Nations Association, and was a fervent supporter of the missionary activity of Methodism. In 1954 he was elected Vice-President of the Methodist Conference and to the end of his life his immaculate, silver-haired figure was familiar in the councils of the Methodist Church

With so many interests it might seem surprising that his paramount concern was with youth, but throughout his life he worked with young people and loved them. This was manifested by the fact that at Muswell Hill in North London, where he lived, he bought a magnificent site—a fine old residence in spacious grounds—and, in 1924, made it available for youth work, conferences, and related activities. In 1947 he gave this North Bank property to the Methodist Church to be used as a youth centre. In it there now stands the headquarters of the Division of Education and Youth of the Methodist Church, and also a students' hostel.

Going too fast?

Up to the 1960s, apart from the first home at Wallington in the outer suburbs, there was no MHA home in London itself. Various suggestions had come to nothing. It was at this period that Richard Connell, who had been a minister in the Highgate circuit and knew Guy Chester well, suggested through mutual friends that he might consider making some part of the North Bank estate available for a home. This he very readily did and, in 1966, The Meadows was opened.

Its exterior is unusual and, at first sight, not specially attractive. But it has been built to fit unobtrusively into its tree-backed setting and from its windows the views are varied—from gardens still full of flowers in the autumn and a tennis court to the Victorian houses of Tottenham or of Muswell Hill. Once inside its advantages are clear, for it has pleasant lounges and the residents' rooms are designed in groups of six to fit round bays where residents can meet by the tea-bars and easily make up companionable morning coffee or afternoon tea gatherings.

The shops are only just outside the gate and the church a few hundred yards away.

At least as important is the closeness of the Chester House youth hostel.

It has been said already that elderly people find youth stimulating and often respond readily to the new contact with the modern world which they introduce. Nowhere is this more true than at Muswell Hill.

On five nights a week they come in to serve evening drinks, and those who move away often maintain the friendships they have made and come back to visit 'their' residents. Muswell Hill church is where these young people mostly worship and their presence there, too, can be a stimulus to those from the home who attend it. But the close proximity of the youth headquarters has added another more long-term youth element to the life of The Meadows. Each year they have found someone from continental Europe to work for twelve months in the home, so that Switzerland, Germany or Scandinavia have become familiar countries to these elderly British residents. Young continental European workers, provided in the same way, are also to be found at Shirley, Wallington and Woking.

'I didn't find it easy to settle down, after living in the Midlands and being part of an active church there', said one new resident. She showed how much the presence of young people could mean. 'But after I'd been here about a month the young people were taking the evening service at the church. They chose "Lord of the dance" as one of the hymns—and came dancing down the aisles while they sang. They drew me out of the seat to join them. Do you know, I began to feel at home at once! It was splendid. And now they've found me a job in the Junior Church—in the Beginners. Young people *do* make life interesting!'

Overseas workers have been employed in nearly all the homes, and they have come from a dozen European countries, from West Africa and America, from the West Indies, South East Asia, Malaysia and Japan. If a list were made it would cover every continent and more than a score of countries.

Richard Connell, the general secretary, got a black eye at Hitchin.

It was nothing to do with the MHA, but he referred to it when Elmside, the new Methodist Home, was opened there in 1966. He had once played cricket for his Luton school against Hitchin Grammar School, he said, and disregarding his captain's advice about where he should stand, had been hit in the eye by a fast ball when he was keeping wicket. The reference was appropriate, for the grammar school's grounds are only divided by a fence from Elmside.

Mr Hubert J. Moss was a well-known provision merchant in Hitchin, and a Methodist. In his later years—he was over ninety when he died—he wanted to benefit Methodism in some way, and he chose to do so by making his house, Elmside, with its extensive ground, available to the MHA at a very concessional price. There was only one limitation; he should live in it until his death. The condition was very readily accepted.

Elmside was in an ideal situation. Its grounds, mainly lawn-like grass, were contiguous with the playing-fields of the grammar school and, farther from the house, with an area of public land known as Butt's Close. Only a very short distance away was a main shopping street of the old town, and a Methodist church stood in it.

But snags soon emerged. The town council was unhappy about the idea of a home. It turned out they thought it was to be for retired ministers—apparently a forbidding prospect—and that local people would have no say in what went on there! Even when this was satisfactorily cleared up another even more awkward matter cropped up. The council wished to compulsorily purchase some of the Elmside ground for a car-park on the main street. Connell stressed the need of quietness for the residents and suggested that they used some of the land at Butt's Close instead. Mr Moss pointed out that this was public land. It belonged to Commoners . . . in the middle ages it had been used for archery and there was a centuries-old charter making it available for two statutory fairs each year.

In the end there was an unusual, but happy, issue. A well-known multiple store wanted to establish a large branch in the town at precisely the same time that the Methodist church ran into harrassing financial difficulties about structural repairs. The multiple store bought the Methodist church, the church bought the ground wanted at Elmside and paid the MHA the same sum that the MHA had paid Mr Moss for the Elmside site. The council agreed that the church should provide a car-park for general use, since it was anxious to have the store in the town. The town had a new store and a rather smaller car-park; the Methodists had excellent new buildings; the residents at Elmside have a church only a little way from their front door. Honour was satisfied, with amenities all round.

Mr Moss's old house became the staff quarters of the new Elmside—and very spacious and attractive accommodation, too. The entrance is through the house, and the incomer has an immediate awareness of space and light. A completely new wing was built for the thirty or more residents, including some double rooms. All the rooms face south and the views are of green lawns, common and playing-fields. By an imaginative piece of design, though the outer wall of the wing runs straight, the corridors curve slowly away as one walks down them, eliminating entirely any institutional look in the long wing.

On some afternoons many of the women residents will be out —at the Women's Fellowship in the church a hundred yards away across the lawn—and there is a strong sense of community between church and home. Before and after meals, as in all the other homes, they lay tables and clear away. But they share more fully in helping the staff in other ways. In some rooms residents are busy sewing and mending—for the house or for other people. A retired minister may be discovered helping one of the younger residential staff who is taking a correspondence course in the Old Testament. The staff speak as affectionately of the residents as the residents do of the staff.

This is a home built for happiness.

13

'Deeply in debt'

Harrogate Flatlets/Cramlington/Norwich/Falmouth

In the first fifteen years every home that was opened, with two exceptions, was already old when it was taken over. They were comfortable-sized private residences; hotels like Tankerton and Leamington; a nursing home at Bath; or houses which had been used as schools, like Bognor and Hathersage. Despite alterations and extensions, and though residents often preferred them to more modern types of building, they were not ideal even when they were re-planned. It was not always easy to provide adequate staff accommodation, and fire precautions were rightly having to conform with higher standards of safety. Extension was sometimes impossible and, in most cases, difficult.

The two exceptions were Woodbank at Woking and Hall Grange at Shirley—one a completely new building and the second a new home attached to the attractive earlier house.

Of the first six houses built in the 1960s four were adaptions or extensions of other buildings. Again, only two were purpose-built—Bury St Edmunds and Scarborough. Of the three mentioned in the previous chapter, two—Wolverhampton and Hitchin—involved very large new buildings, though the earlier house remained in use, and Muswell Hill was a new building.

By contrast, in the case of the three homes in this present chapter, all were completely new buildings and the architects were commissioned to provide, as far as might be possible within a limited budget, exactly what was needed in such a home. A great deal had already been learned, both from adaptions and from new purpose-built homes. The costs would be high, but at that point it seemed that the advantages would be with homes designed for their specific purpose. With only two exceptions, Lincoln and Ipswich, this would be the policy until, at any rate, the period at which this book ends. And, by the time the three homes were opened in 1966 others were already being planned, sites inspected or negotiations in progress.

But, by then, another need was becoming evident.

Those who had served the MHA longest as officers, and who had seen the development of the homes, had always been aware of how much a 'good' home depended on the staff, and particularly on the matron. Conditions of work were congenial and rewarding, but with recurrent shortages of staff, they were always arduous. Yet many, especially the matrons who had given longest service, were prepared to work until they could go on no longer. Richard Connell and his colleagues were increasingly uneasy because they found senior residential staff working harder than they ought and, at the same time, showing signs of real strain.

The reason was occasionally, though not always openly, admitted. They had to prove to themselves, as well as to others, that they were fit to go on working because the alternatives might be frightening. What would happen to them when they came to the end of their service? Not old enough to enter one of the homes, and not always wanting to do so, they frequently had no home of their own and, in some cases, no close family to whom they could turn. Their case, indeed, though they were a younger generation, was parallel to that which had stirred Walter Hall to strive towards the creation of homes for the elderly in 1937 and during the war.

Yet one surely did not begin yet a second group of homes for retiring staff?

At the same time it had to be admitted that the MHA was deeply in debt . . . not in terms of finance, but of obligation. So was Methodism as a whole and especially the residents of the homes over a period of twenty years. *They were in debt to devoted women who were not likely to press their case.*

Reg Spray and his wife were made sharply aware of the problem when they visited one of the homes and found the matron's health giving real cause for concern. She admitted that one of the reasons was anxiety about her own future. It was in the week following this visit, while they were still talking about the situation, that there came an offer of long-term significance. Professor Richardson, living in Harrogate, made a tentative offer to the

MHA of his own home. It was next door to Berwick Grange, the second home to have been opened and in many ways one of the most attractive.

The natural response would have been to buy it as an extension to Berwick Grange. But Connell and Spray had other ideas. With the ready assistance of Fred Kettlewell, the Harrogate treasurer, careful inspections, assessments and plans were made. Sir George Martin and Mrs Lang, who shared Connell's concern for retiring staff, supported his scheme. The general secretary, however, was a very shrewd man. He suggested to the committee a variety of uses for the new house—and in each case indicated the problems that such use would create. It was only when they were wondering if the offer should really be accepted after all that he spoke of his own heartfelt hope—that the house might provide flatlets for retired staff, and especially those who had served as matrons.

In the event, Kettlewell Court—converted into six flatlets—was opened by the wife of a famous Leeds medical personality, Sir Ronald Tunbridge, themselves loyal Methodists. The opening was on 6th July 1967—the twenty-first anniversary of the opening of Berwick Grange itself. By the date of the official opening the first residents were in occupation of the flatlets.

Other flatlets and accommodation of this kind were to follow in several places, most of them on grounds already occupied by the MHA homes.

Retired staff in the flatlets willingly accept that in return for accommodation they should serve for brief periods, health permitting, when the need for relief staff arises. Thus, because there are constant vacancies in the homes owing to sickness, retirement or resignation, or even because new staff for new homes has not been recruited, many of the retired staff find themselves in their old rewarding work from time to time. Such opportunities are exhilarating. They make new friendships and renew old ones; they are able to offer wise counsel when their advice is sought; without them many of the homes would have been in desperate straits.

The contribution of retired staff has been invaluable. It is no exaggeration that some homes might have had to close if they had been unable or unwilling to fill the gaps. They have done far beyond what was or could be expected of them.

Once Kettlewell Court had been established its value was immediately apparent. A gift of £20,000 from the Joseph Rank Benevolent Trust was made available for a block of flatlets at Bexhill when that home was being planned. When the home at Poole was being built a small house on the site was retained for the same purpose. Much more recently a gift from Mr and Mrs W. K. Wilson of Sheffield has made it possible to provide similar accommodation at Scarborough. In the grounds of Willersley House, Hull, Ivy Cottage and the Lodge have been recently modernized for the same purpose. Other accommodation will undoubtedly follow, in new or adapted premises.

Problems which some people feared might emerge by having retired staff adjacent to the homes have never arisen. The tenants of the flats have enough in common, and sufficient variety of experience, to provide interest and stimulus. Above all, they have proved a base from which retired staff can go back to temporary work and still retain the security of a home of their own until—as many undoubtedly will—they themselves become residents in the homes they so obviously love.

Kettlewell Court was well named. Fred Kettlewell, M.A., with Sir George Martin and Mrs Lang, is one of the veterans of the MHA. A well-known businessman of Harrogate—his father was a station-master in East Yorkshire—and closely connected with Wesley Chapel, he was a key figure in the early days of the organization. Other local treasurers, too, can trace their association with MHA to the opening of the home they serve, but Fred Kettlewell was the treasurer of the second home to be opened. He took up his duties in 1946, and only retired, old in years but not in mind or interest, in 1969. By that time he had been appointed treasurer for the new retired-staff house which was named after him.

It would be difficult to over-estimate his contribution. Unlike Sir George Martin (who sought his advice gladly and regularly) or Mrs Lang, who were national figures in Methodism and exercised considerable authority in the committee, Fred Kettlewell worked almost behind the scenes. But he was one of the architects of the early days and helped to build a strong organization out of simple and tentative beginnings. Not least was his importance seen in the advice he gave to new treasurers about their duties and the way he 'coached' them to be expert in administration and in helping the residents. The counsel he gave to others was more than matched by the loving care he gave to residents and staff in Harrogate.

One of the three new homes opened in 1969 was the 'farthest north' yet. This was at Cramlington in Northumberland.

Newcastle upon Tyne, with London and Bristol, was one of three focal points of Methodism in Wesley's day and the base he maintained for his work in the north. Here in 1746 he established the 'Orphan House', at once a preaching-house, a residence for the local 'minister', a Sunday-school and a hostel for travelling preachers. Throughout the district, and in the fell country, are evidences of Methodist penetration in Wesley's own time, while Newcastle itself was always a Methodist stronghold. Here in the north-east, especially amongst the miners, Methodism played a key role in the foundation of the early trades unions. Within the area there are today strong and community-minded churches. Yet, despite this inheritance. the nearest MHA home was at Scarborough.

It was the Rev. Arthur Jex, superintendent of the Whitley Bay circuit, who turned wishful thinking into action. When he approached the office at Westminster the reply was predictable. 'Find a site and we'll look at it!'

Another millionaire now comes into the story—though no man looks less like one. William Leech had little to boast about in the 1930s except initiative and foresight. But, coming from a 'working-class background', he believed in 'working-class people'. Given a chance to break out of their restricted existence and the depressed areas in which they lived, he knew they could and would make good in new surroundings. The heart of the problem, for many of them, was the lack of good housing which they could afford.

It may have been business shrewdness which led him to buy

some land before the last world war. It may have been the accident of war itself which prevented his developing it and building on it until the war was over, when its value had risen astronomically. It may have been good business sense which turned a small building site, over the years, into the first of the large housing estates in the north-east. No one would question the driving, far-sighted ability which made him one of the wealthiest property developers of the region. But it is also beyond argument that throughout his career he has had in mind provision and benefit for the sort of people from whom he came.

This has been manifested in the way his wealth has been used. A very small man in physique, quiet and shy in disposition, he is a philanthropist of the most open-hearted kind. Amongst other things, for instance, he set up a trust to benefit a group of five charities—one of them the Methodist Missionary Society—which makes available to each of them income of nearly £100,000 a year.

It was to William Leech that Arthur Jex went with his idea of a home for the aged. Leech, at this point, was engaged in the creation of a completely new town, Cramlington, and he listened with interest.

He told Jex of a possible plot of ground. 'There's a lot of old junk on it, but it might do. I'll give it to you if it's what you want.'

On the site there now stands the splendid Cramlington home. It was opened by Mrs Mary Trembath, niece of Mrs Lang, who was eventually to take over her office as treasurer of the MHA, and was named Harwood Court in honour of Sybil Haddock—known to generations of *Methodist Recorder* readers as Margaret Harwood.

Purpose-built, the home is surrounded by the typical, smallish houses of which Cramlington is mainly comprised. Those who live there are, generally, young people with families and the sound of children's voices is seldom unheard for long. The lawn is good but not too large. There is a covered patio, where flowers bloom from spring to autumn. Though the shops are some distance away there is a bus stop outside the home and, while some residents choose to use it, others are still content and able to walk when they go out. The church is perhaps half a mile away and, for those who need it, church members with cars provide transport as is the case with all the homes.

Of the thirty-one residents only three are men. One of the limitations which all homes have to accept is the small number of men compared with women residents. More men would mean a greater variety of interest and more stimulus—but women on the waiting-lists greatly outnumber men, as they do in the homes themselves. The men at Harwood Court at any rate have one 'privilege' to which they hold firmly. Though the places in the dining-room are changed regularly (as they are in many of the homes) the three men are allowed to keep a table for themselves!

There was by this time a better 'spread' of homes about the country. Every main area, though not every Methodist district, had one or more. There was still pressure to open in Cornwall and South Wales, and the Midlands with its heavily-concentrated population had only Wolverhampton, since Leicester was specifically for those needing extra care and attention. For new homes there were plenty of suggestions, but many turned out to be unsuitable for a variety of reasons. It was nevertheless, to many people, something of a surprise that another home should be opened in East Anglia, a fairly sparsely-populated area with few lateral rail-links. As in many cases it was the result of a suggestion by a layman who had access to the ear of the committee.

At this time the Rev. Reginald W. Hopper, B.D.—who was in 1975 to become the Pastoral Director of the MHA—was superintendent minister in Norwich. William Trower, a director of a firm of local building contractors, was a leading layman in the city, a 'Conference-type' of Methodist who was influential in the East Anglia district. Like Reg Hopper, who was a member of the executive committee, he appreciated the work of the MHA.

'Would you be interested in a useful site for a home in Norwich?' asked Trower.

The question was followed by a visit to an empty site behind the houses on the Ipswich road, which belonged to a fellow director of John Young Ltd, the builders. The place was no more than a paddock, and a donkey munched away at the grass as they walked round it. Its advantages were patent. It was secluded, but just off a main road. There was plenty of space for planning a completely new home, and room for an adequate garden which would have no awkward slopes or rises. A bus-stop was nearby. The more the officers thought about it the more suitable it seemed to have a home in Norwich. It was a lovely and busy city, steeped in history, a county capital, but one in which land was scarce, and the site was approved and bought.

In April 1969 Cromwell House was opened. The two-storey building is widely spread and makes an imaginative use of the site, forming three sides of a square. Within the square, and beyond it, are delightful gardens. There is ample parking space, as well as garages—a feature which not all the homes possess. In the wide hall is a fish tank, its gaily-coloured tropical occupants providing a focal view-point, and near by are shelves of books regularly changed by the library.

Cromwell House has two notable features. The first is its dining-room on the first floor, so that no cooking smells from the adjoining kitchen reach the lounge on the ground floor. The other, a complete innovation in its time, was not achieved without controversy.

It had always been the practice of the MHA to provide wash-basins in each bed-sitting-room. This helped to make the rooms both private and personal. But Reg Hopper, with knowledge of other homes run by voluntary societies and local authorities, and knowing how much older people wish to preserve their personal dignity, felt strongly that something further was needed. Why should the rooms not be so designed that each resident had a personal toilet?

The ensuing tussle in the executive committee was sharp. There was already a critical feeling that the newer homes were moving beyond 'comfort' to 'luxury'. Indeed, Sir George had expressed himself as shocked and angry when local press reports had described newly opened homes as 'luxurious' in their fittings and furniture. There were others who agreed, though the general secretary insisted that good furnishings were less expensive in the long run than cheaper ones which would have to be renewed more quickly. The argument was that there now appeared to be a very different approach from the early days when 'economy' was the yard-stick of expenditure. Surely, even though the elderly were accustomed to higher standards in their own homes than they had been in the 1940s, 'private toilets' were a highly questionable extravagance.

Hopper won the day, but he recognized that other people might adopt the same attitude. What, indeed, would be the stance of the local authorities? When the medical officer of health and the deputy welfare officer from the Norwich City Council came to inspect the home he was ready for what they might think—but not for what they actually said.

'This is splendid . . . real foresight . . . you've saved yourselves 75 per cent of the trouble that, in our experience, arises in old people's homes!'

Norwich had established a pattern that was to be generally followed in all the new MHA homes.

Few places in the country could be farther from Cramlington, or more different in location from most of the homes, than Falmouth. It was here, at last, that Cornwall had its first home.

Richard Connell had visited the county, at the invitation of the district chairman, early in the 1960s. The gap between that date and 1969, when the home was opened, well illustrates not only the time-lag but the thorough-going process of viewing, assessing and selecting between a first concept and the finished home. On that first visit he examined three sites between St Austell and Truro; three in Falmouth; three in Truro; and several on the way back to the county border. Of them all, Falmouth appeared the most attractive town, and a site belonging to the Earl of Kimberley the most suitable place.

Until the time of Charles II the name of the tiny town at the edge of the water was Pennycomequick, which has nothing to do with the financial expertise of its citizens but, in the Old Cornish language, meant 'the village at the head of the valley'. It was changed to Falmouth—the town at the mouth of the river Fal—by Charles II, who gave it its charter in recognition of its loyalty to the Royalist cause in the Civil War. The setting is splendid by any standards. On the edge of the English Channel, secluded from the north gales of Cornwall's north coast, it has a magnificent harbour, sheltered by the peninsula on which stands Pendennis Castle. The Carrick roads beyond the harbour are a maze of creeks and inlets. It was said that a hundred ships of sail could anchor in them without the masts of any one of them being visible to any of the rest.

It was here that Robin Knox-Johnson ended his lonely 'round the world' voyage. More than three centuries earlier Sir Walter Raleigh ended his voyage round the world here, too. On the night Raleigh came ashore he was feted at Arwenack House, the home of the magnificent and sometimes notorious Killgrews. Winston Graham's *Grove of Eagles*, an outstanding historical novel, tells their story, with Arwenack House as its principal setting.

It was in the grounds of the old Arwenack House that Langholme, the Falmouth branch of the MHA, was built.

The original mansion had been pulled down and rebuilt by Squire Wodehouse of Norfolk, whose descendants were to become Earls of Kimberley and give their name to the South African diamond-mining township. It was the Earl's agent who was prepared to negotiate the sale of the land and, a little later, made the overgrown garden round the ruins of Arwenack House available, too, thus offering direct access from Langholme to the main street by the harbour below.

But even when the site was chosen there remained the need of money.

In 1955 Captain T. B. Clarke, who had been Commodore Captain of the Sheaf Steamship Company of South Shields, and who later moved to Falmouth, left a sum of money to the MHA. He hoped that it might be used for a home in Cornwall and it was set aside for that purpose.

Much later, Mr Harold Edmunds, of Sutton, in Surrey, visited the head office at his own request and met Reg Spray. Before they had coffee he handed over a tightly-rolled piece of paper, about the size of a cigarette, which he withdrew from his waistcoat pocket. It proved to be a cheque for £10,000.

Startled, Spray asked him: 'Are there any strings attached to this?'

'No', answered Mr Edmunds. 'I would only say that I am a

Cornishman.' The implication was clear and these two gifts were the foundation of the Falmouth home. It was completed early in 1969.

The house is delightful—airy, light and with an appearance of space. An open staircase from the large foyer leads to open landings above. The lounges are on the first, not the ground, floor and thus have extensive views of the docks and the harbour beyond the ruins of Arwenack House. There is a pleasant water-garden and pool in the patio which is visible from the entrance and the hall.

It is not surprising that the residents are happy here. The main street is easily accessible through the gardens. The church is near and, each fortnight during the winter months, transfers its evening service to Langholme. The residents work for their own sale —and recently gave 50 per cent of the proceeds to the general funds of the MHA and the other half to be divided between the National Children's Home and the Methodist Relief Fund.

This Falmouth home must be the only one that has had two openings. It was due to be opened in February and, though it seemed early in the year, the London officers had no doubt about Cornish weather. Falmouth would be very pleasant at that time of the year. But Cornwall is not England—and, though Falmouth was unaffected, England was snowbound on the day of the opening. Lord Rank, the official opener, was snowed up, and so was his sister Mrs Lang. Sir George Martin was feet deep in snow in Leeds. London was cut off from Cornwall. But the Sprays arrived by train, and so did Sidney Hall, the association's solicitor and one of the founder's sons.

What should be done?

The schoolmaster-treasurer spent a morning telephoning official guests with a 'snow in England' warning, and cancelling the official opening. Meanwhile, preparations went ahead for those who would come in any case. With over eighty people present on the landings and in the hall Reg Spray and the treasurer made their unofficial speeches, Sidney Hall spoke informally about his father, and the 'irregular' opening was carried through to everyone's satisfaction.

It was June of that year before the 'proper' opening took place and a plaque was unveiled.

> 'This home is named Langholme in honour of Mrs Hilda Bartlett Lang who, from the beginning of the Methodist Homes for the Aged in 1943 in the dark days of the war, inspired the work. In company with Sir George Martin (Chairman) and the Rev. Walter Hall (Secretary) she brought wise judgement and loving kindness to this service for God. For more than 25 years she has held the office of Honorary Treasurer, and continues to serve with distinction.'

The plaque is dated February 1963. Apart from that questionable inaccuracy it says nothing which is not abundantly true.

In the days that followed Falmouth heard of Langholme year by year. The handyman-gardener made the first garden a joy and then transformed the wilderness round Arwenack House. One year Falmouth tied with Aberdeen for the first place in the 'Britain in Bloom' competition. Langholme won the prize for the best-laid-out garden that year, as it had done in the two previous years. Under the gardener's skilled hand and eye it won three more prizes in other years, too. In the hall five certificates and three statuettes pay tribute to his work.

The 1970s

Mature and established residence

'The old haven't only seen and heard it all before—they have survived and triumphed through it.'

'You don't *grow* old; when you cease to grow you *are* old.'

14

High rise

Bexhill/Bowdon/Poole

One thousand two hundred years ago King Offa of Mercia—Offa's Dyke in the Downs behind Hastings preserves his name—gave a charter to build a church on England's south coast. Four centuries later the Normans landed not far away and conquered the Saxons at the battle of Hastings. The Saxon manor was taken over by the Normans. It went to the Sackville family in Queen Elizabeth's day and, in the nineteenth century, passed by marriage to the De La Warr family. It was the 7th Earl who developed a seaside resort round the site of the ancient Saxon church.

Bexhill, as it became, near neighbour of St Leonard's and much older Hastings, is a quiet resort favoured by quiet and often by elderly people. A good many retire here.

One of those who made his home at Bexhill-on-Sea was Dr Leslie Weatherhead, famous preacher and best-selling writer, former minister of the City Temple but by love and loyalty still a Methodist. It was he, more than anyone else, who saw Bexhill as an ideal spot for a Methodist home. Though it was an estate agent who found the site it was Leslie Weatherhead who advocated it.

Now, a long double-storey building, Richmond, stands there. With five immense windows in the lounge/dining-room facing on to the beautifully maintained lawn, its lines are gracious and promise comfort within. Its design is contemporary, with features the MHA had generally adopted. There is a spacious hall, with bright pictures, flowers and a bookcase. The rooms all have personal toilets. Grouped on four corridors, with tea-bays and comfortable chairs, the residents enjoy feeling that they belong to smaller manageable communities within a larger whole. The lift—a 'must' in all the homes—is the gift of Dr Weatherhead in memory of his wife.

Richmond is closely linked with its local church and circuit. The local social committee is active, sharing in coffee mornings, outings and 'the sale'—from which profits go partly to the amenities fund and partly to charities such as the Methodist Relief Fund and the District Benevolent Fund. 'We've been helped ourselves through this lovely house, so we want to help others', is the general attitude.

From its upstairs windows Richmond overlooks a lovely sixteenth-century cottage next door, and not far away is the sea. The residents thrive in the good air—and so do the flowers and the beds of heather.

It was in 1968, when Richmond was first planned, that the Joseph Rank Benevolent Fund gave £20,000 to build flatlets for retired staff at Bexhill. Named Colley Corner, in memory of Joseph Rank's home near Redhill, they were opened in 1971, the same year as Richmond itself. Each of the six flatlets, modern in design, has a lounge/living-room, kitchen, bedroom and bathroom. As from the other 'retirement flatlets' the workers return gladly to take stand-in duties in any of the homes where need arises—though not in the home by which they live.

In 1968 The Joseph Rank Benevolent Trust made what is, at present, its last 'challenge offer'. It was larger than any that had gone before. There would be £25,000 a year for three years for each £25,000 raised by the MHA itself. It was a generous offer, and effective.

A second home was also opened in 1971. This was at Bowdon, at Altrincham in Cheshire.

The legal requirements governing the establishment of a nursing-home are very strict and, despite many enquiries—almost entreaties—which reached the head office on behalf of those needing such a home, it is clearly beyond the scope of the MHA to provide them. But the 'special homes' at Bath, Leicester, Hull and Woking have the full approval of the medical officers for health and of the welfare authorities. It seemed opportune to establish another such home—and so Handsworth, at Bowdon, came into existence. A generous legacy from the estate of Miss

Olier helped considerably in the purchase of the site from the Earl of Stamford.

There was one major difficulty. The site, in a quiet residential area on a tree-lined road, was very limited. Indeed, it seemed impossible to spread sufficiently widely to house an economic number of people. There *was* a solution, suggested the architects, but it was novel and startling. 'If you can't build outwards, build upwards!' The committee had more reservations than the architects. Would not elderly people, all of them frail, find it disturbing to be on the third floor, even if the fourth were reserved for the staff?

Surprisingly, they find it interesting and exciting.

Next door is a block of 'luxury flats'—'and ours is much nicer', assert the Handsworth residents. Instead of the flat facing of contemporary architecture, the home has bays of large-paned windows rising from ground to roof. Its yellowish brick seems to promise warmth and comfort. From the big windows, where the tea-bars are set, there are views of nearby houses and gardens, and the tree-shaded road with a school not far away. 'It's lovely when the mothers come to fetch the children . . . just when we're having tea . . . it's like the grand prix.'

Possibly the mothers might not appreciate the tribute to their driving but it indicates that these shut-in elderly people are not really shut in at all. 'Grand prix racing' may be a thrill they enjoy by proxy, but so are football and athletics, show-jumping and moorland walks, mountaineering and state occasions. Through the boon of television those who can seldom go out find their way into the outside world. Sports and cowboy films, thrillers and variety all have their addicts—sometimes rather surprising ones—though for many the Sunday evening religious programmes are the highlight of their viewing.

One of the newer innovations in all the homes is that, while most residents have long had their own radios, a growing number in these days have their small personal television sets in their own rooms, too. Some matrons see this as a threat to community life; others, more realistic, accept that it is something which makes a room even more one's own private home.

How do residents in these homes for the frail spend their time? They have their own pattern of life.

'We have breakfast at 9.0—not too early; then back to our rooms to tidy them up. There's tea at the tea-bar in the middle of the morning. And we can go and visit our friends in their rooms, or invite them to ours. We always have a rest after lunch. And after a cup of tea we go to the lounge . . . oh, yes, there's TV, of course—but we read, or do a bit of sewing . . . and a bit of mending . . . and a bit of chatting. It's surprising how quickly it's bedtime!'

Commendation from the residents was mirrored by something more official when the town clerk of Manchester wrote after visiting the home. '. . . the complete absence of anything approaching institutionalism . . . informality . . . the whole atmosphere was one of homely contentment and satisfaction.'

It is equally matched by the matron's comment. 'I've never enjoyed a job so much. It isn't like work at all!'

But at this period in the early 1970s this new home was not the only thing to be 'rising high'. Costs were rising quickly, too —and higher.

The cost of Ilkley, with its original extensions, had been £30,000. That was in the late 1940s. In the early 1960s Bury St Edmunds had cost £78,000—and that was a completely new home. At the very end of the 1960s Norwich cost almost double—£134,000. Within three years of the opening of the Bowdon home the new home at Nottingham would cost £247,000. Less than two years afterwards, in 1975–6, the home at Southport would need some £300,000.

Nor was it merely the price of a new building that was eating up money.

By the 1970s older homes were a drain on resources. There had to be renewals and repairs. Kitchen facilities, sometimes out of date, needed replacing. Staff accommodation had to be replanned and extended to meet the proper requirements of residential workers. There were homes where staff had to share the same toilets and bathrooms as residents—and both found it embarrassing. There were homes where even the matron had little privacy and less room. To recruit staff would increasingly involve the MHA in offering accommodation, individually and in terms of staff-rooms, which matched that provided by other welfare organizations and local authorities. Day staff could go back to their own homes, but for the residential staff 'home' was where they were—and it was common justice that it should not be inferior. If 'homeliness' and 'comfort' were criteria for the residents—and this had been so from the beginning—those who gave them such loving, and sometimes sacrificial, service deserved no less.

But all this cost money. At Glen Rosa the new lift, together with additional accommodation for staff, an improved kitchen and dining-room and a sun-room, cost £69,000—more than double the original price of the house.

Fortunately there was a 'high rise' in income, too.

By 1970 the general income (excluding residents' payments) had touched £280,000, including legacy income of £181,000. Both the Flower Fund and Margaret Harwood's Christmas Appeal in the *Methodist Recorder* brought useful contributions. But it was the wide variety of appeals stemming from the facile imagination of Norman Spencer which kept the MHA before an increasingly wide public. In 1968 there had appeared a fascinating, if expensive, brochure, *Homing*, broken down for local use into regional handouts. This not only illustrated the homes themselves, region by region, but many of the Methodist associations—most of them little-known—were pictured, too. Few productions in Methodism have been more attractive, or more interesting.

From 1960 an annual event had been the publication of a special 'Christmas appeal' by a public figure. Produced as a small leaflet for general distribution, this was also featured in the religious and national press. The first half-dozen were by well-known Methodists—Selwyn Lloyd, Donald Soper, Sir Hugh Foot amongst them—but other names, still more widely known, followed them year by year. Mrs Harold Wilson, Colin Morris, David Frost and Derek Nimmo were only a few who were prepared to lend their public image to a genuine plea for support. Alan Watson, TV commentator and son of the manse, made a nation-wide impact with a Panarama interview with three old ladies in Blackburn. The following year he was the 'personality' featured in the Christmas appeal leaflet based on facts from the TV interview.

But perhaps the most effective innovation was the 'Solicitors' Portfolio'—containing information, brochures and leaflets about the MHA—which was sent to all solicitors in Britain, and kept up year by year with new material. It was Mrs Spray, wife of the administrative officer, who promised to address some 8,000 envelopes to solicitors. It should not take many weeks . . . or months . . . of her spare time. But the months grew longer, for the list of solicitors turned out eventually to have 23,000 names on it! This mammoth task was all done at the Sprays' home in Woking and the envelopes despatched from Woodbank, the Woking home.

Of its effectiveness there can be no doubt whatever for, year by year, the legacy list grew larger as interested solicitors suggested the MHA as a worthy cause which donors might include in their wills.

It is noteworthy that, for many years, the printing for the MHA has been done by Mr Peter Frost, of Clifford Frost of Wimbledon, a Methodist family which has given fine and immaculate service in this way.

William Stoate, the second honorary general secretary, eventually retired to Bournemouth and it was his great desire to have a home at Poole, not far away. From time to time he would phone Richard Connell about yet another site of which he had heard. None proved suitable. Hotels and houses all had to be turned down in a wide area round Bournemouth through problems of price, planning permission or general desirability. Poole was a place where many people wanted to go, as well as the MHA, and house prices reflected its popularity.

The Maidments were traditional Methodists of Poole, loyal and generous without holding office. George Maidment had established a business which included public works and roads, and his son, George Frederick, extended it into civil engineering and long-distance road transport. Both father and son were married, but G.F. was without children. Both were anxious to do something that would benefit the community through their estates, though the legacies might well be long delayed. Their principal wish was to establish a home for elderly people.

Their solicitor, John Miller, was a Methodist who was to become Vice-President of the Conference in 1973, and through him they learned something of the work of the MHA. After making provision for their wives, both father and son willed substantial legacies to the MHA. There was no stipulation about Poole, but their solicitor had no doubt about their preferences.

Then suddenly G. F. Maidment, the son, died—a few months before his father. Unexpectedly and sadly, after considerable legal and fiscal problems had been sorted out, the MHA had funds to provide a home in Poole.

At that juncture a group of houses became available on Parkstone road. All four of them, adjacent to each other, were purchased. Today, Maidment Court stands in memory of warm-hearted Poole Methodists, in one of the most desirable situations that could be found. All the residents' rooms face the front, looking over Parkstone road to a wide and fascinating vista. Beyond the park is the sea-water lake, with children's boating; behind it the railway runs into Poole; beyond that is the sweep of Parkstone Bay. Sandbanks, at one end of the panorama, and Brownsea Island at the other, are more distant prospects and the Lilliput Yacht Club, opened by round-the-world local yachtsman Sir Alec Rose, provides a constant flow of boats and interest.

Maidment Court was opened in 1972 by Sir Keith Joseph, then Secretary of State for Social Services. He described it as of 'five star quality'. But it is the quality of life, rather than its design or amenities, which makes it what it is—a true home and a happy one. William Stoate, who had pressed the MHA to open a home in Poole, was its first resident. He lived out his last days, and died, here.

But if life is meant to be enjoyed, death is not a terror.

It is perhaps at this point, more than any other, that homes such as this are distinguishable from those run on a secular basis. In many local authority homes for the elderly the matron is reticent about reporting a death. 'It upsets people!' But the matron at Maidment Court had other views. 'I tell them when someone is ill, and I tell them at once when someone has died. People here are not afraid of death, or worried when other people die. This is the true mark of their Christian faith.'

'Methodists', said John Wesley, 'live well and die well.' This still remains true.

Even so, deaths are infrequent. Contented people tend to live long, as well as happily. In 1971 there were only eighty-eight vacancies in twenty-nine homes—and this was about average. The opening of Maidment Court took in another thirty people—but it still left some 900 or more on the waiting-lists.

15

Royal Event

Lincoln/Penarth/Stratford-on-Avon/Nottingham

The north country local paper had a picture of an elderly woman being hugged by three children. 'Saying good-bye to Auntie' was the caption. 'She has lived in the same house for almost eighty years,' ran the story, 'seeing the neighbourhood go down and down. The chapel up the street has been her life, but even there it's not the same. Her friends have mostly gone—some dead, some to live with their families. For Mary, unmarried, the neighbours' children have been her family. But now she is going, too—to a lovely home by the sea. Run by the Methodist Homes for the Aged, she knows she will be happy there.

' "It's wonderful", says Mary. "I thought the day would never come. They've had my name down on the list for four years—and I've kept on wondering if I would ever get there while I was fit enough to enjoy it".'

Mary is only one amongst many who wonder the same thing. With a waiting-list which now has 1,000 names, it is not surprising. But there could easily be a great many more. It was recently reported that there are 9 million people of retirement age in Britain—and 2 million of them are living alone.

What is the position? In what ways, if any, has the policy changed since the early days of the MHA?

It must be remembered that when Walter Hall persuaded the Conference to establish the Methodist Homes for the Aged he had no thought of providing for more than a few of those who might wish to come. Nor had he any conception of the flood of requests he would receive. With only half a dozen places in the first home at Wallington there were thirty times that number who enquired, and many were pitiable in the extreme. Today, though there are 1,000 names on the waiting-lists there are more than 1,000 residents in the homes.

In fact, there are two 'waiting-lists'—and considerably more hope than in the early days. A small leaflet, *20 Questions and Answers*, provides a good deal of information for those who 'want to know'.

It will be helpful, perhaps, to include a measure of relevant information here.

The homes are intended for the aged and lonely people of Britain.

While they primarily exist for Methodists, others are gladly welcomed if they are 'kindred spirits'. Members of other churches are to be found in most of the homes and, in any case, financial support is by no means exclusively from Methodism.

To accept active people in their early seventies, however desirable as a way of bringing vitality in the homes, would prejudice the chances of older people whose names have been on the waiting lists for some considerable time. In practice most are nearer eighty—or over—when they are admitted.

There are two waiting-lists. The B List consists of those whose needs are not immediate, while the A List consists of more urgent cases awaiting admission.

People do not age as quickly as they did in the 1940s and 1950s. They are more anxious to maintain their own homes, and better able to look after themselves, than used to be the case. State pensions and assistance also make this easier. As a result names are not now accepted for the wiating-list until the age of seventy.

While applicants may state a preference for a particular home, available vacancies in that home may be few and long delayed. It makes admission more speedy if the preferences are not too specific.

Residents contribute according to their means, both income and capital being taken into consideration. But money matters are discussed only between the applicant and the head office. Though treasurers receive the residents' payments, matrons do not know—and would not wish to know—what individual residents pay. All pensioners retain a certain amount of their pension—and this, in any case, is required by law.

Many of the other questions will be answered on the leaflet, or by correspondence.

Lincolnshire has always been a place of pilgrimage for Methodists, and especially for Americans. Epworth was John Wesley's birthplace and the Old Rectory, where he grew up, is a part of Methodist history. Tourists go to Lincoln to see the cathedral with its twin figures of St Hugh, the great bishop-builder, and the swineherd who brought a gift for its building, on the pinnacles above the carved west front. Not so many who glance at the castle by the cathedral recall that John Wesley's father, the scholarly but improvident rector of Epworth, was imprisoned here for debt.

Probably fewer still climb, or even go down, Steep Hill and notice the old houses which belong to Christ's Hospital.

Some four miles from the cathedral, deep in the country, lived Henry Stone, Lord of the Manor of Skellingthorpe, until his death in 1693. He bequeathed the manor to Christ's Hospital, in London, including the farms called Decoy, Lounds and Stone's Place. The *Stones Arms Inn* and memorials in the parish church at Skellingthorpe preserve the family name and memory. So does the manor house—Stones Place—which was built in 1812 on the site of Henry Stone's seventeenth-century farmhouse. A plaque on the side of the house records the names of the president, treasurer and clerk of the charity.

This house, acquired by Lord Liverpool after retiring as Governor-General of New Zealand, passed from owner to owner for a century and a half. There is a record of a Methodist society meeting in the drawing-room in the middle of the last century. Much more recently it became an officers' convalescent home, a prisoner-of-war camp and a NAAFI centre with nissen huts amongst the trees and rose-beds. Overgrown and shrouded with shrubs and creeping plants, the brick foundations and walls of the nissen huts still remain.

It was to this house that Philip Race, a Lincoln solicitor who had been very active in the early days of the Methodist Association of Youth Clubs and had been the youngest Vice-President of the Conference, drew the attention of Richard Connell. It was for sale. Would it not make a highly attractive Methodist home?

Set amongst eight and a half acres of woodlands and gardens, filled in spring with daffodils and narcissi, with a large vegetable garden, fish-ponds and lily-ponds, lawns for croquet and putting, it retained the air of its original manorial glory, though much would have to be restored in the garden and the house, as usual, would need considerable extension. By the summer of 1972 Stones Place at Skellingthorpe was ready for opening. Two new wings flanked the old house, built with the same sand-coloured stone to more or less the height of the original house which formed its centre-piece. The first residents had been in occupation, as usual, for some months before the official opening.

8th June 1972 was a great occasion for the MHA. It was the birthday of Her Royal Highness the Duchess of Kent—and on this highly personal day the Duchess came to open Stones Place. Closely connected with the organization 'Age Concern' she could well appreciate the values that lay behind the gay, sunny, informal occasion. Her charm, as well as her informed comments and her thoughtful interest in the life of the residents, made her presence endearing and her visit memorable.

Stones Place is an attractive place to visit, but here—as in all the homes—it is made plain that this *is* a home, not a tourist centre, and that its residents are not show-pieces. There was once a coach party which arrived at the door of one of the homes, unloaded and thronged round the entrance. To the matron they announced: 'We've come to look round!' But they were not admitted. Parties need to make prior arrangement if they wish to visit homes and at Stones Place residents entertain small groups to tea in the dining-room, half a dozen or so to a table while they act as hostesses. If they are willing to open their rooms to visitors, the residents leave their doors open. If not, they retain their privacy behind closed doors. 'You can't just have your home invaded when you don't feel up to seeing visitors', summed up one busy, elderly lady on behalf of all her friends.

In 1972 those associated with the MHA rejoiced in the distinction which was given to Richard Connell. In that year he was awarded the M.B.E. in the Honours List. Rightly, he insisted that it was not merely a personal honour but a public tribute to the work of the Methodist Homes for the Aged for almost thirty years of active service to the community.

In that same year Sir George Martin made an unusual and splendidly open-handed gift to the MHA. This was Scruton Farm, near Northallerton. Valued at some £72,000 it stands as one of the capital assets of the MHA, an out-of-the-ordinary holding for a charity of this kind which is unlikely to depreciate in value. It was yet one more assurance that the chairman did not only rejoice in the past work of the organization but had a very strong belief in its future.

The MHA hit the headlines at the Methodist Conference in 1973. It had less than its usual friendly reception, and some of its careful planning was completely upset.

There were two pieces of business on the agenda which were of interest to Conference members.

The previous year a suggestion had been received by the Conference that the MHA be asked to consider providing Sheltered Housing for the elderly who did not yet need the full provision of the homes. The committee considered the matter and reported that it would be wrong to divert its resources from the tasks committed to it when the MHA was founded. There was no dissension about this, and attention was concentrated on another, and more thorny, subject.

Both Richard Connell and Reg Spray had decided a year earlier that they ought to retire in 1973. Accordingly a minister, Deryck Howarth from Peterborough, had been nominated to the 1972 Conference to take over as general secretary in 1973. But this was a period when there was a severe shortage of ministers in the circuits. All districts had had to reduce their strength by one minister and, in some cases, by more. The district synods, during the year, had expressed their minds unmistakably. In effect, they said: 'The MHA has managed with a supernumerary (that is, retired) minister for almost thirty years . . . why should they want to change now, when the circuits are short of ministers?' To explain to the Conference how greatly the work had grown was pointless. They already knew, and had made up their minds. The nomination was rejected. In effect, this meant that a minister in the 'active work' could not then or, presumably, later be appointed general secretary of the MHA. Richard Connell and Reg Spray returned to their work at the head office and to constant itineration round the country at a time when both would readily have retired. It was 'back to square one', and both were to work as hard as they had ever done before they finally retired two years later.

The Conference decision was plain. If the MHA wanted a secretary younger than the average active supernumerary minister it would have to be a layman.

The search began.

More than two years passed, after the opening of the Poole home and the royal event at Lincoln, before another home was opened. Even then, though the home was ready to receive residents, the opening was delayed to ensure that the fire precautions were acceptable to the authorities. A tragic fire at an old people's home in Nottingham had shocked the nation and drawn attention to the deficiencies which might be present even in well-planned buildings. The lessons of that disaster have been taken to heart throughout the country. Old people are less able to help themselves than most others, and a thoroughgoing examination of all homes, whatever their ownership, has been conducted. Extensive work on additional fire-precautions has been carried out in all MHA homes.

At last, in December 1974, came the opening of Morel Court in Penarth—the first and long-awaited home in South Wales.

The decision to establish a home in the area was by no means a sudden one. The general secretary had earlier discussed the possibility with Maldwyn Edwards, chairman of the Cardiff and Swansea District. Sites had been examined near the coast and inland but the objections were the usual ones—too far from shops and church, gradients too steep for elderly people to negotiate.

The Gibbs family have long been active in the Penarth area. Their personal interest and generosity has been shown in the provision or support of significant community work—Headlands Community Home, where the National Children's Home cared for over fifty disturbed boys and girls; Ardwyn, at Dinas Powys, another NCH home; the Youth and Community Centre, Kynance, at Dinas Powys; and the creation of flats for retired ministers. Dr John Gibbs, an ex-Vice-President of the Conference had made ground available for Methodist International House, a striking high-rise building near the sea. Both John Gibbs and his wife Sheila had felt it would be undesirable to concentrate too many Methodist institutions in Penarth, but after all the other possibilities had proved unsuitable they very readily offered part of their own garden to the MHA.

It was accepted with enthusiasm.

Morel Court is near to the sea. Indeed, it is possible to 'walk round the block' to the sea-front and back without crossing a road. There are seats by the roadside and on the sea-front. Though the shops are a quarter of an hour's walk away there is a bus-stop outside the house. Residents are reasonably mobile and active, and the setting is a considerable attraction. So is the roof space for sitting out in sunny weather, with shelter from the prevailing winds. This last has been included in many of the newer homes.

In terms of staff accommodation, however, Morel Court took a significant step forward. Residential staff are essential, but to insist in the cases of matrons that 'only unmarried women need apply' seemed likely to cut off very valuable sources of supply. Morel Court, therefore, included a 'family flat' for the matron which, as it turned out, was exactly what was needed.

Throughout Britain, and indeed throughout the world, the cost of living went on escalating to an alarming degree in the early 1970s, and even more steeply towards the beginning of the decade. In the same way building, maintenance and ordinary housekeeping bills were a source of anxiety with which both the head office and local homes found it had to cope. Residents' payments did not keep local homes solvent and end-of-the-year rescue operations from the head office were not abnormal. New bulding, renewals and extensions and day-to-day running were all competitive claims on income. It was a matter of thankfulness, therefore, that the general and legacy income continued to rise. In addition, however, there was in 1973 a very large gift from Lord

Rank, then in his eightieth year but still very closely in touch with Methodism.

The gift was £100,000.

In view of the inhibiting effect of rising costs it was a matter for rejoicing that the next home to come on to the MHA lists was already a 'going concern'.

Edward Youell had grown up as a poor boy in Coventry. His mother died when he was very young, and he could always remember a day when his father showed him his open hand with a single penny in it. It was all they possessed. Born towards the end of the last century he grew up in a world where struggle was familiar and where initiative, personal courage and toughness often counted for more than advantage of birth. He found his way into the building industry and, by the beginning of World War II, was well established. Indeed, his reputation stood so high that he was very much engaged in the rebuilding of Coventry, which had been so appallingly blitzed during the war. His personal fortune continued to accumulate and, like many men of his type, he was anxious to use some of it to benefit others.

Retired to Stratford, he decided to do something for the elderly people of the town. A Methodist himself, and knowing something of its work, he consulted the MHA about the sort of place old people would want to live in. The result was a home that approximated closely to the current concepts of MHA design.

Youell bought Rowley House, just off the Warwick road, built a number of good bungalows in the ground which sloped below the main house, and added to the main house a large wing with the sort of accommodation which would be found in most of the newer MHA homes.

From the lounge, which is on the main floor of the old house, the immediate view stretches across the river Avon to the Shakespeare Memorial Theatre, with a glimpse of Shakespeare's statue by the bridge. The more distant prospect beyond the town is of the hills, and a quiet vista of the Warwickshire countryside. Built for local people, many of them semi-professional, the residents have a continuing interest in the affairs of the town and the district.

It was this home, Cedar Lawn, which Edward Youell passed over, complete and fully running and in occupation, to the MHA in January 1975.

By this time both 'Father' Connell and Reg Spray could see retirement in sight. Both planned to leave the MHA in the summer of 1975 and, by now, their succession was assured. In curious fashion, the refusal of the Conference to appoint a minister in the full-time work to follow Connell in 1973 had actually established the future.

Since Spray had also intended to retire that year, and a layman would be needed to take over his work as administrator, an advertisement had been published offering 'one of the most exciting jobs in Methodism'. It neither mentioned the MHA nor used its address. A number of people replied. Amongst them were Ron Sellars and Brian Callin.

Brian Callin, M.A., B.Sc., was a son of the manse who worked first as a research scientist with Shell and then moved to its personnel side. He became personnel manager at the research laboratories in Egham, Surrey, in 1970. Much involved in youth work, he and his wife Joan found an additional interest in the care of the aged, and helped to run an old people's sheltered housing project in Chester. Now living at Woking, and more from curiosity than conviction, he replied to the advertisement. He said that he would not be available for three years, knowing that no organization could afford to wait so long however qualified the applicant might be.

The Callins were fellow-members with the Sprays at Trinity Methodist Church in Woking. Indeed, Mrs Callin had said to her husband on one occasion: 'Wouldn't it be splendid if you could get a job like Mr Spray's with the Methodist Homes!'

No one could have been more surprised, therefore, when the Sprays came up to them one morning after service. Reg had his familiar twinkle when he spoke, in his rather dry voice. 'We were interested to get your application!'

In the event, another applicant, Ron Sellars, was taken on the strength of the MHA immediately as estates manager, a new but very necessary appointment. The readiness of both Connell and

Spray to continue until 1975 made it possible to plan for Brian Callin's appointment in that year as the chief officer of the MHA.

Ronald Sellars, with a B.Sc. in engineering, was closely associated with his local church and, like Callin, had a special interest in youth work. After two years with Surrey County Council he had served under the Methodist Missionary Society in Rhodesia from 1952–65. First as a technical officer at Waddilove teacher training institute and then for two years as head of the science department at Tegwani training institute, he had moved to Moleli secondary school which he took two years to build and then served as principal for a further three. Returning to Britain he worked as a lecturer and then set up his own surveying consultancy practice. With a life-time of practical knowledge in construction, design and maintenance, as well as purchase and sale, his application in fact underlined the need for the full use of these skills in the growing organization. It was a new appointment but a very necessary one.

Brian Callin would bring initiative, compassion and valuable experience to his work as secretary. But, at the same time, it still seemed essential to have a minister within the MHA. Pastoral care had been proved to be of great importance to the residents and perhaps even more to the staff of the homes. Fortunately a minister was becoming a supernumerary in 1975 who had had a wide-ranging ministry, both as a missionary and a garrison chaplain in India and within the British circuits. He had knowledge of other homes outside Methodism, as well as being a member of the executive committee of the MHA. The Rev. Reginald W. Hopper, B.D. had been closely connected with the creation of the Norwich home and was at that point at Harrogate—again with close links with Fred Ketterwell, the veteran treasurer, and with Berwick Grange and the staff flatlets. He agreed to serve for a period from 1975 as pastoral director.

But another change, this time within the Methodist constitution, brought yet another new situation. The restructuring of the many Methodist departments into seven divisions resulted in the Methodist Homes for the Aged becoming a constituent element in the Division of Social Responsibility, until then the Christian Citizenship Department. This was agreed by the Conference 'on the explicit understanding that the MHA will continue to operate as a distinct and largely autonomous organization'. Brian Callin became a secretary of the new division.

One more home was to be opened before the two chief officers retired. This was at Nottingham.

Queenswood, at Chilwell, near Beeston, set among modern houses with a primary school at the back where its grassy playing-fields bring young life right up to the boundary of the home, is as attractive as any of the MHA homes. One of the comments of the general secretary in the 1950s was that he could never be sure which was the more important to old people—the matron or the cook! Neither appointment, in experience, is easy to fill adequately. Queenswood has good food, warmth, space, community life, privacy—and loving care. Reasonably near to small shops, there is a car-service to take residents to the church at Beeston, some little distance away. As in most of the newer homes there are double—or rather twin—rooms for husband and wife, though they can if necessary be turned into normal 'singles'.

True, the residents have hardly had time to settle into anything like a traditional routine, but like everywhere else, they already find plenty to occupy themselves. But it is atmosphere which counts as much as activity.

'. . . . and there's such an atmosphere of contentment and relaxation and happiness . . . so much sense that this is "home" . . .'

One resident's words after a few months at Queenswood speak for all.

The staff quarters here are notably good. Like those at Penarth they begin to create a pattern for the future. Yet, unfortunately, it is still true that Queenswood could have been opened several months earlier if a matron had been available. Constant and widespread advertising, as well as personal commendation, were strangely ineffective. Though the home was more or less ready when Morel Court was opened in January 1975 it was not until June that the official opening took place.

The need for staff is paramount in this work. The lack of it is the greatest headache, and indeed heartache, which the head office and the local committees have to face.

By the spring of 1975 there were thirty-three homes in existence, all of them happy, comfortable, rewarding places in which to work.

But, at that time, there were thirty residential staff needed, many of them senior and responsible positions.

16

View from '75

Jersey/Southport/Ipswich/East Kilbride

Only one more home was to be opened in 1975 and that was tenuously, rather than intimately, connected with the MHA.

Alexander Kilham, one of John Wesley's preachers who later founded the Methodist New Connexion in 1797, preached in Jersey in 1784. These island people had no liking for an English Methodist, and a mob interrupted his sermon with mud, stones and dirt. But Methodism won its way, and established itself as a part of island life. Today, near the site of Le Chapelle de Pas, where Kilham preached, stands Maison La Cordiere—Rope Walk House—the purpose-built Jersey Methodist Home for the Aged.

The home is the fulfilment of a dream which began to take shape when the first donation was received towards the end of 1963. A legacy from Miss Amy Noel boosted the fund. In 1965, to comply with legal requirements in the Channel Islands, a limited liability company—Methodist Homes for the Aged (Jersey) Limited—was registered, and the search for a site began. Advice from London (though the home must belong to Jersey and could never be linked with the MHA in Britain) was sought and accepted. A new home, not an old building adapted, was desirable. Indeed Richard Connell, visiting the island, pointed out an excellent site as he walked round the perimeter of Fort Regent. It was not, however, for sale. Then came an anonymous donation of £8,000, enough to begin negotiations for the site. An appeal for £150,000 had to be stepped up to £200,000 because of escalating costs, and then again by another 10 per cent. But the money came.

Corresponding to the best designs of the British homes, Maison La Cordiere was opened on Maundy Thursday, in March 1975, by E. F. C. Ereaut, Esquire, the Bailiff of Jersey, and dedicated by the President of the Conference, the Rev. J. Russell Pope.

The sponsorship of the home is Methodist but gifts have come from all quarters and residence is not restricted to Methodists, though only those with a residential qualification under Jersey Housing Regulations may be admitted. While the MHA did not in any way beget Maison La Cordiere, there is a strong family relationship.

As this book is being written other homes are either being built, are on the drawing-board or are in negotiation stages.

One will be opened before this account appears in print—Connell Court at Southport, in Lancashire. On the Ainsdale side of the town, not far from shops or sea, it is a four-storey brick building, its exterior made interesting by bays rising from ground to roof. As a result, each resident's room has a large window which offers extra space and light.

Ground is already in the possession of the MHA at East Kilbride, the new town to the south-east of Glasgow, which will accommodate the first MHA home in Scotland.

On the secretary's desk, or in his files, are suggestions for advance into other parts of the country. But undoubtedly the most appealing and human story behind any of the new homes comes from Ipswich.

Mrs Elsie Hill was a member of the very first MHA committee. Keenly interested in the overseas mission of the church, especially in women's work, she never allowed concern for those who were far away to blind her to the needs of those around her. It was an attitude shared to the full by her husband. Dr Arthur Hill—a gentle, gracious man known as 'Uncle Arthur' to innumerable people in Ipswich—had been a GP but finally became the senior surgeon at the Ipswich and East Suffolk Hospital. For many years respected for his services in Methodism, he would certainly have been Vice-President of the Conference if he had not been so heavily committed to other activities. He acted as a kind of 'honorary medical consultant and adviser' to the MHA. The Hills' home in Ipswich was seldom empty of guests and visitors, many of them ministers invited 'for a rest' after illness, and it had its own pervading atmosphere of hospitable affection.

It was perhaps not surprising that, after Elsie Hill died, Dr Hill should offer his house, now too large for his own needs, to the MHA. It was bought at a very concessional price. There would have to be considerable extensions, and these might raise building and planning problems, but no house would have more love in it.

Just at this point another distinguished Ipswich resident comes into the story. The Rt Rev. Leslie Brown, Bishop of St Edmondsbury and Ipswich, lived in the same road as the Hills. They were friends, as well as neighbours, and the Bishop had a long-standing affection for Methodism. He had been known to invite himself to the local Methodist house-group by merely knocking on the door and asking if he could come! It was when Leslie Brown was having coffee with Arthur Hill that the doctor posed his question.

'Wouldn't you rather live here than in your big bishop's house?'

'You know I would. I've always loved your house.'

'Then couldn't we come to an arrangement? Make *your* house available to the MHA, and you have this one instead.'

To neither of them did the idea seem audacious. Within forty-eight hours the Church Commissioners were on the phone to Dr Hill.

To a comment, made later, that this was a very warm-hearted thing to do for Methodism the Bishop made a simple reply. 'But I *am* a Methodist . . . and a Presbyterian and a Congregationalist . . . as well as an Anglican. I am a presbyter of the Church of South India.' No one would have imagined that church union in South India would have had so direct a bearing on the Methodist Homes for the Aged in Britain.

Much more remains to be done, but it is hoped that in the much larger bishop's house—neither 'palace' nor 'Lord Bishop' for Dr Brown—Methodists will find a home with the same atmosphere of gracious affection that there would have been in Elsie Hill's home in Ipswich.

Behind the Ipswich home lies easily the largest single gift ever made to the MHA. This is an immensely generous donation of £200,000 from the 'Norwood Trust' in memory of Mr Thomas England. It was Mr England who 'discovered' the Alexandra

Hotel in Dovercourt, and Mrs England is a member of the Dovercourt Committee. However 'concessional' the price of an actual house there are, in these days, very costly building operations and alterations, as well as costly equipment such as lifts and kitchen furnishings, which must be met.

One question is bound to be asked. Will the MHA be extended as quickly and widely in the future as in the 1960s and the early 1970s? Many associated questions have to be answered. If new homes do not appear to spring up all over the country at the same rate it will not be because the MHA officers and committee are unaware of the need or indifferent to the waiting-list. But it may well be that, once more, it is time to assess what has already been achieved, continue to examine in detail the necessity for repair, renewal and extension (all costing a great deal of money at current prices) and, above all, set as one main priority the needs of residential staff for fuller amenities and, in some cases, more realistic accommodation.

It is beyond question that those on whose shoulders and hearts rest the responsibility for thirty-four homes, with more to come, and the needs of a large number of elderly and aged people who hope to find a place in them, have the same deep concern as that which stirred Walter Hall's compassionate heart before the homes came into existence at all.

On 25th September 1975, there was a historic gathering in the lower rooms of the Westminster Central Hall. The staff of the MHA, members of its committees, local treasurers, colleagues in other divisions situated at Westminster, were meeting to say 'farewell'. There had been changes, all coming at the same moment at the end of the Methodist year, which were startling in their range. Sir George Martin, in his nineties, had ceased to be chairman after thirty years of indefatiguable leadership and high vision, and had handed over to John Miller, who had helped to bring the Poole home into existence. The deputy chairman, a new appointment, would be Derek Lyons, a knowledgable and well-travelled businessman with an Irish accent who had given valuable service in the Redhill circuit. Mrs Hilda Bartlett Lang, too frail to attend the gathering, had passed on the office of treasurer to her niece, Mrs Mary Trembath, who had acted as her assistant for some time. She too had held office since the inception of the MHA, matching great personal generosity, always unpublicized, with a detailed examination of every piece of expenditure, however small, and always interpreting 'pounds' in terms of 'people'. Richard Connell and Reg Spray, both able to retire at last, found Brian Callin and Reg Hopper in their old offices and were well content after jointly spending some forty years in adminstration, travel, committees and, above all, in personal thought for those in the homes. Miss Lena Picking, her own memory retracing the years to the days when Walter Hall began it all, was retiring after twenty-eight years.

There were few speeches at this gathering, and those that were made were brief. There were presentations of affection and goodwill . . . it must have been the only time that, in a meeting connected with what had once been known as the Temperance Department, a retiring chairman was presented with a silver-plated ice-bucket!

More than anything else, there was talk . . .

. . . and the stirring of memory.

Looking back over those thirty years, what had been achieved?

Thirty-four homes had been opened, or were in process of construction.

Twenty-five Methodist districts had one or more homes within them. Of the rest, two were island districts, Shetland and the Isle Isle of Man; one was the Welsh district, Cwmry; one, the Channel Islands, had its own home.

The cost of building had risen from £30,000 in the 1940s to some £300,000 at Southport.

The income, too, had risen prodigiously. In 1950 the general income had been £47,000; in 1975 it was £720,000, including £25,000 from the 'Rank Challenge offer' and two gifts towards purchase of two homes totalling £98,000. Legacies, reported with the general income, had risen from £5,000 in 1950 to £416,000. The Flower Fund was £11,500. Residents payments were £600,000 and income from local authorities £80,000. Against all this the total running of the homes had been £860,000.

In terms of money, there had been some spectacularly generous gifts and support through the years.

The Joseph Rank Benevolent Trust had contributed nearly a quarter of a million pounds, much of it 'challenge offers' which stimulated other giving. The 'Norwood Trust' gift of £200,000 was the largest single gift, and Lord Rank had donated £100,000. Sir George had handed over his farm, valued at £70,000. There had, indeed, been half a dozen millionaires who featured in the story. In addition, there had been many cases of property made available for use or development at very much under-the-market-value prices.

Yet, when all that is said, the steady flow of support has come through small gifts, some from churches or circuits, most of it from individuals. It is because of this that the work has continued, for it symbolizes a deep quality of concern amongst ordinary people. Certainly these givers were in the minds of some at that farewell gathering. Reg Spray, for instance, would remember opening a small packet with twenty pound notes in it, and an anonymous note of good wishes in elderly handwriting. And he would not forget the resident who had 'little to bless herself with' but, every time there was a rise in her pension, sent it quietly to the head office.

But, even with such awareness as that, the MHA cannot rate money first. What has counted more than anything else in 'the real building of real homes' has been service and love—never to be assessed in terms of pounds and pence. From the staff of the homes, from local committees and local churches, from boys and girls and young people, a torrent of affection has been poured into the homes which has helped to make them utterly different from almost any others.

It would be unjust not to recall others who have contributed to this work. Amongst them the architects stand high. Such homes cannot be created by the adaptation of a single, simple blueprint. They are only achieved by imaginative thought by those who design them. In some cases, though not in all, the architects have had Methodist associations, or have been closely involved in church life. They include Highet and Phillips of Guildford; Building Design Partnership, arising from the firm of Grenfell, Baines and Hargreaves; Bernard Blanchard and Gerry Frankish, of Hull; Leslie Buxton; Beresford Smith; and Alick Gavin. Homes of many kinds had been visited, residents and staff questioned, earlier inadequacies reconsidered and, every time, some new improvement suggested. Expertise had been closely linked with understanding.

There have been few references to the local authorities in this book, mainly for want of space, but the head office and the local treasurers would speak with great respect about the representatives of local and statutory authorities. They have seldom been less than helpful and, in many cases, have been generous in consideration, suggestions and colleagueship.

The official Home Committees, meeting twice a year but giving service for the whole time, and the local groups who have supported the staff, worked with matrons, visited and cared for residents and raised both interest and money, have been indispensable fellow-workers with the head office. It is largely due to them that interest in the MHA has not only been sustained but widened through the years, inside and outside Methodism.

Above all, those who realized how and why the whole organisation of the MHA worked so effectively had in mind the debt that was owed to the local treasurers—laymen and retired ministers who gave so much of their time to their local homes. Many of them were at that farewell gathering.

Yet, when all was said, done and remembered, the unseen people who really crowded that downstairs room at Westminster in September were the hundreds of men and women who daily gave thanks to God for the inspired leadership and courage that brought the MHA into existence . . . the residents of the homes themselves.

More than a thousand of them, mainly in their eighties, many in their nineties, a few past their century, have a rich, full and friendly life which was unthinkable in the 'workhouse days' of the 1930s. They go shopping or to clubs or to church when they might well have imagined themselves beyond such activities. They make furniture and tapestries; they paint pictures or go bird-watching; they play classics on the piano or croquet on the lawn;

they take up flower-arrangement or work out the crossword or the chess problem in the daily paper; they worship together or drink tea together; they make blankets for refugees, raise money for charity. They are very human. Sometimes co-operative, sometimes awkward, they may be the life and soul of the company, or shun company altogether. They may find faith easy, or confess that they have never been free from doubts. They may be gay, or withdrawn from long anxiety; full of concern for others or mainly interested in themselves.

They are as far from the Bognor journalists's sentimental picture of the 'dear little old lady' as it is possible to be.

But, men or women, frail or busy, whatever they do or cannot do—they *live*.

Life of this quality, communal but private, stimulating but restful, undergirt by security and surrounded by love, is the great gift which the Methodist Homes for the Aged have been able to offer to growing numbers of people throughout the past thirty years. In an age when the elderly live on to become old in ever-larger numbers, when the norm in a family is likely to be four generations rather than three, and when the greatest threat to the old is not ill-health but loneliness, it is important that this work should be supported to the full.

The next best thing to home, for the elderly, is 'home from home'.

Official opening dates, names and addresses

1945 *Ryelands*, 15 Beddington Gardens, Wallington, Surrey SM6 0JF

1946 *Berwick Grange*, 5 Otley Road, Harrogate, North Yorkshire

1946 *Cliff Dene*, 11 Marine Parade, Tankerton, Kent

1947 *Glen Rosa*, 24 Grove Road, Ilkley LS29 9AW

1948 *Greenways*, 225 Hawthorn Road, Bognor Regis, West Sussex PO21 2UW

1948 *19 Fulwood Park*, Liverpool L17 5AD

1949 *Moorland House*, Station Road, Hathersage, Sheffield S30 1DD

1950 *Stratton House*, 16 Park Lane, Bath, Avon BA1 2XH

1951 *Homewood*, 19 Kenilworth Road, Leamington Spa, Warwickshire

1952 *Woodbank*, Holly Bank Road, Hook Heath, Woking, Surrey GU22 0JP

1953 *Moreton*, 13 Drakes Avenue, Exmouth, Devon EX8 4AA

1955 *Astoria*, 30 Llannerch Road West, Colwyn Bay LL28 4AS

1957 *Starr Hills*, Ansdell Road South, Ansdell, Lytham St Annes FY8 5PQ

1958 *Hall Grange*, Shirley Church Road, Croydon, Surrey CR9 5AL

1962 *Alexandra House*, Marine Parade, Dovercourt, Essex CO12 3JY

1962 *The Martins*, Vinefields, Bury St Edmunds, Suffolk IP33 1YA

1963 *Aigburth*, Manor Road, Oadby, Leicester

1963 *Willersley House*, 85 Main Street, Willerby, Hull HU10 6BY

1963 *Green Meadows*, Colwell Road, Freshwater, Isle of Wight PO40 9SN

1963 *Priceholme*, Givendale Road, North Leas Avenue, Scarborough, Yorkshire

1966 *Elmside*, Elmside Walk, Hitchin, Hertfordshire SG5 1HD

1966 *The Meadow*, Meadow Drive, Muswell Hill, London N10 1PL

1966 *Engelberg*, Ash Hill, Compton, Wolverhampton, Staffordshire

1969 *Harwood Court*, Highburn, Cramlington, Northumberland NE23 6AZ

1969 *Langholme*, Arwenack Avenue, Falmouth, Cornwall

1969 *Cromwell House*, Cecil Road, Norwich, Norfolk NR1 2QL

1970 *Richmond*, Collington Lane East, Bexhill-on-Sea, East Sussex TN39 3RJ

1971 *Handsworth*, West Road, Bowdon, Cheshire WA14 2LA

1972 *Stones Place*, Skellingthorpe Road, Lincoln LN6 0PA

1972 *Maidment Court*, 47 Parkstone Road, Poole, Dorset BH15 2NX

1975 *Morel Court*, Raisdale Road, Penarth, Glamorgan CF6 2BN

1975 *Cedar Lawn*, Cedar Close, Welcombe Road, Stratford-upon-Avon, Warwickshire

1975 *Queenswood*, Cliff Grove Avenue, Beeston, Nottingham NG9 4DP

1976 *Connell Court*, 22/24 Weld Road, Southport, Merseyside

Enquiries

about the work of the MHA should be sent to:

The Methodist Homes for the Aged
1 Central Buildings, Westminster, London SW1H 9NH

Staff

The work of the MHA is dependent on its being able to staff its homes fully. There is a constant need of residential staff who have a genuine love and understanding of elderly people. In some homes nursing qualifications are needed.

If you are interested in this work please address your letter to The Secretary at the above address.